Estrogen

Edited by Wahid Ali Khan

Published in London, United Kingdom

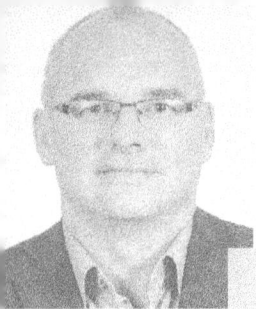
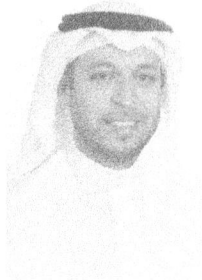
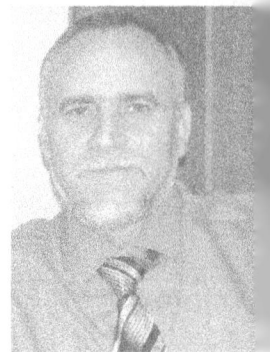
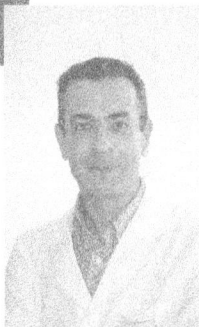
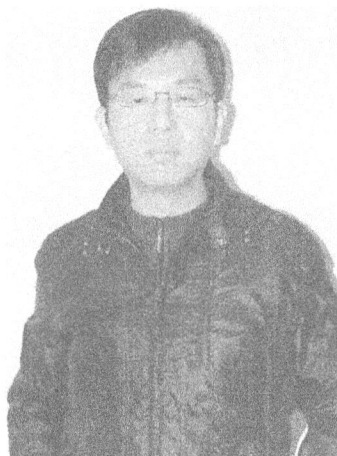
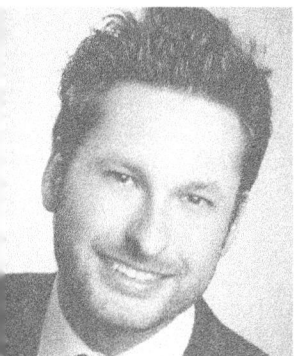
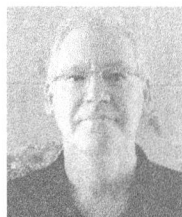

IntechOpen

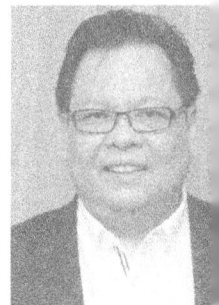
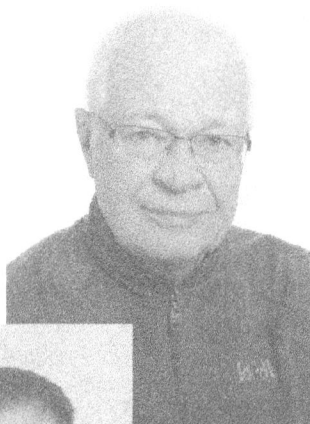
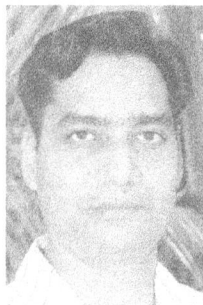
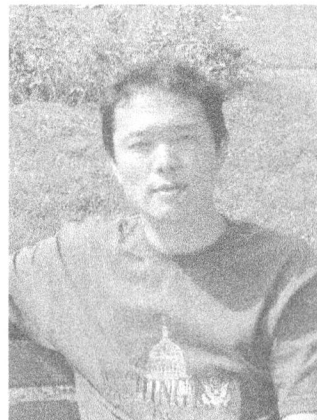
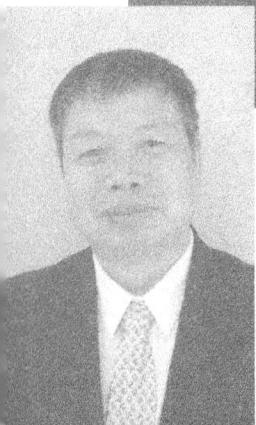
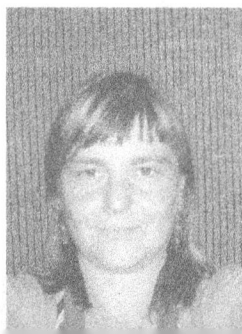

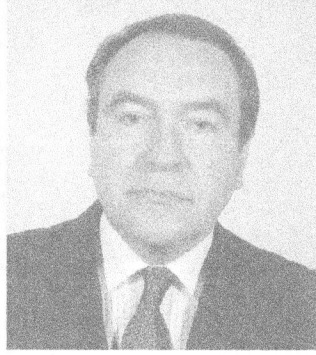

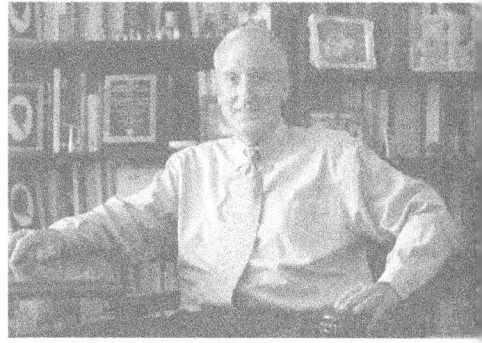

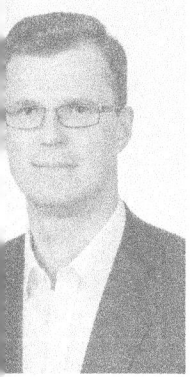

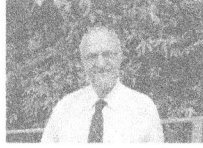

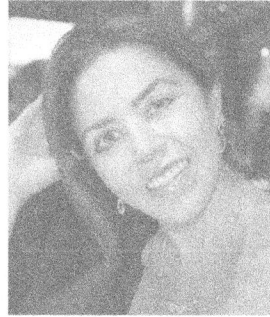

Supporting open minds since 2005

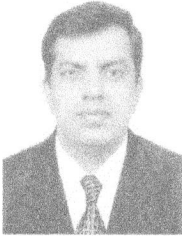

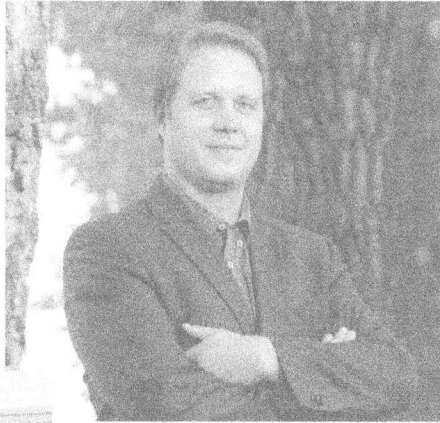

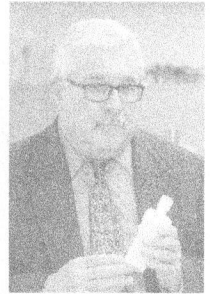

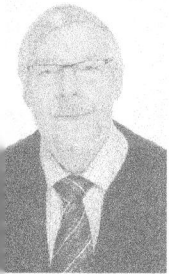

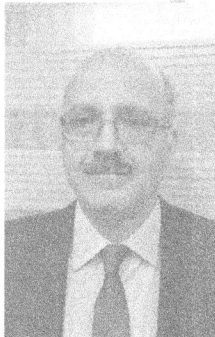

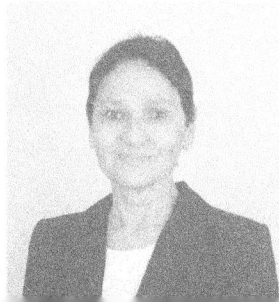

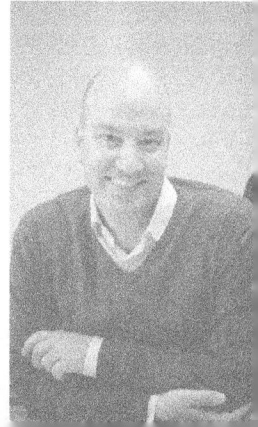

Estrogen
http://dx.doi.org/10.5772/intechopen.73419
Edited by Wahid Ali Khan

Contributors

Joselin Calderón, Carlos Santos, Chun Hei Antonio Cheung, Shang-Hung Chen, Tomoya Kataoka, Kazunori Kimura, Lucija Peterlin Mašič, Darja Gramec Skledar, Manuel Cortés, Salvador Espino Y Sosa, Jacobo Alejandro Gomez-Rico, Myriam Cortes-Fuentes

Notice
Statements and opinions expressed in the chapters are these of the individual contributors and not necessarily those of the editors or publisher. No responsibility is accepted for the accuracy of information contained in the published chapters. The publisher assumes no responsibility for any damage or injury to persons or property arising out of the use of any materials, instructions, methods or ideas contained in the book.

First published in London, United Kingdom, 2019 by IntechOpen
IntechOpen is the global imprint of INTECHOPEN LIMITED, registered in England and Wales, registration number: 11086078, The Shard, 25th floor, 32 London Bridge Street London, SE19SG – United Kingdom
Printed in Croatia

British Library Cataloguing-in-Publication Data
A catalogue record for this book is available from the British Library

Additional hard and PDF copies can be obtained from orders@intechopen.com

Estrogen
Edited by Wahid Ali Khan
p. cm.
Print ISBN 978-1-83880-866-2
Online ISBN 978-1-83880-867-9
eBook (PDF) ISBN 978-1-83880-868-6

We are IntechOpen,
the world's leading publisher of
Open Access books
Built by scientists, for scientists

4,200+
Open access books available

116,000+
International authors and editors

125M+
Downloads

Our authors are among the

151
Countries delivered to

Top 1%
most cited scientists

12.2%
Contributors from top 500 universities

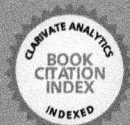

Interested in publishing with us?
Contact book.department@intechopen.com

Numbers displayed above are based on latest data collected.
For more information visit www.intechopen.com

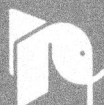

Meet the editor

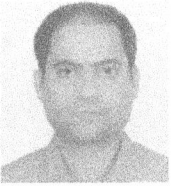

Dr. Wahid Ali Khan is an Assistant Professor in the Department of Clinical Biochemistry, College of Medicine, King Khalid University, Abha, KSA. He has served as a member of the editorial board of more than six international journals and has been a guest editor on two journals. His research interest includes the role of estrogen and its metabolites in various autoimmune diseases. He is also interested in cloning of interferon alpha 2b and discovering its role in the pathogenesis of different types of autoimmune diseases. Dr. Khan has published more than 25 articles, 4 reviews, and 6 book chapters. He is the editor of five books, which have been well recognized and documented within the international research community.

Contents

Preface

The book "Estrogen" has been edited to present the latest topics on estrogen's function and use as a therapeutic agent. Thousands of functions are carried out by estrogen; a few need to be better explained vis-à-vis their proper physiological function. The collection of topics in this book aims to fulfill this need.

Dr. Wahid Ali Khan
Assistant Professor,
Clinical Biochemistry,
College of Medicine,
King Khalid University,
Abha, KSA

Chapter 1

Challenges in Treating Estrogen Receptor-Positive Breast Cancer

Shang-Hung Chen and Chun Hei Antonio Cheung

Abstract

Despite hormone therapy is widely used (as both adjuvant and neoadjuvant therapy) for the treatment of estrogen receptor-positive (ER⁺) breast cancer and patients receiving hormone therapy often show satisfactory initial response, resistance to selective estrogen modulators and aromatase inhibitors is frequently found in patients after prolonged treatment. In this chapter, we will discuss the molecular mechanisms of action of various hormone therapy agents and the biology behind the induction of hormone therapy resistance in ER⁺ breast cancer cells. Recent development of novel agents that can be used to treat ER⁺ hormone therapy-resistant breast cancer will also be discussed in this chapter.

Keywords: aromatase inhibitors, breast cancer, estrogen receptor, hormone therapy resistance, tamoxifen

1. Introduction

Breast cancer is the most common malignant disease and leading cause of cancer-related death for women worldwide. Among all subtypes, estrogen receptor-positive (ER⁺, i.e. expressing estrogen receptors endogenously) breast cancer is the most prevalent type, accounting for approximately 75% of all patients. In clinical situations, hormone therapy targeting the estrogen (ER)-estrogen response element (ERE)-regulated cell survival-signaling pathway is commonly used for the management of ER⁺ breast cancer. The goals of applying systemic hormone therapy in patients with breast cancers are different in separate disease stages and generally hormone therapy can be given to patients with early disease prior to surgery (i.e. neoadjuvant therapy) or after surgery (i.e. adjuvant treatment), and patients with metastatic disease. There are four major classes of hormone therapy agents currently used for the management of ER⁺ breast cancer and they are: selective estrogen receptor modulators (SERMs), aromatase inhibitors (AIs), selective estrogen receptor down-regulators (SERDs), and luteinizing hormone-releasing hormone analogs (LHRH analogs). Even though these agents are all functioned in interfering with the hormone-dependent cell survival-signaling pathways in breast cancer cells, their mechanisms of action are completely different (**Figure 1**).

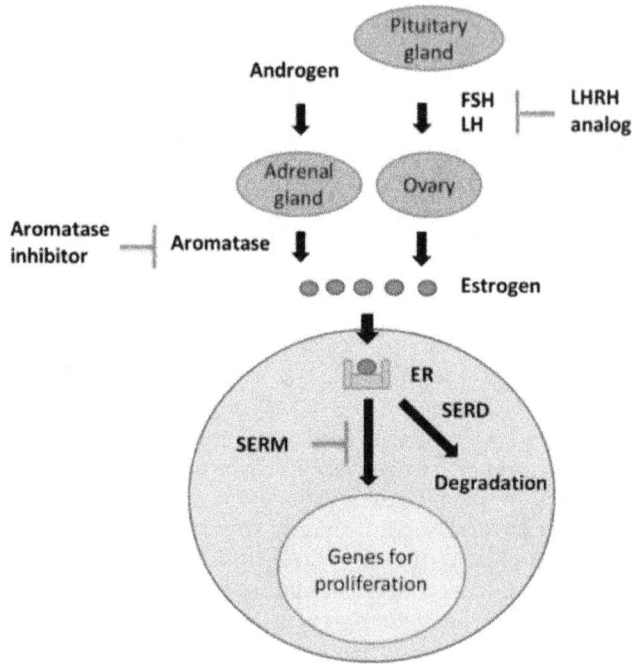

Figure 1.
*Mechanisms of action of different hormone therapy agents like SERMs, SERDs, AIs, and LHRH analogs.
Hormones shown in this picture: follicle-stimulating hormone (FSH) and luteinizing hormone (LH).*

2. Human breast cancer

2.1 Clinical classifications of human breast cancer

Breast cancer is now recognized as a group of diseases with distinct histopatho-logical and biological characteristics. In the last decade, there is accumulating evidence indicating that individualized therapeutic strategies should be applied to treat breast cancers with different expression levels of histopathological biomark-ers which own their unique biological behaviors and treatment responses [1–3]. Currently, the most determinant and commonly used molecular markers in clinical classifications of breast cancers are ER, progesterone receptor (PR), human epider-mal growth factor receptor 2 (HER2), and Ki67. The prognoses and most beneficial treatments of patients would be best evaluated after comprehensive examinations on the expression levels of these molecular markers in tumor cells. In addition to conventional risk factors such as tumor size, numbers of lymph node metastasis, surgical margin with tumor involvement, and tumor differentiation grade, the abovementioned molecular biomarkers have to be included in a modern pathologi-cal report of breast cancer. Breast cancer classification based on expression levels of these four biomarkers are summarized in **Table 1**.

Immunohistochemical (IHC) staining is the most accepted and widely used method to determine the expression levels of these biomarkers (i.e. ER, PR, HER2, and Ki67) clinically. Based on St. Gallen Consensus 2009 [4], ER+ and PR+ tumors were defined as if 1% or more immuno-reactive cells were identified. Noticeably, the definite percentage of breast cancer cells displaying nuclear immuno-reactivity for ER and PR must be reported, because the higher numbers of positive cells indicates the larger anticipated benefit of hormone treatment.

Subtype	Molecular profile
Luminal A	ER$^+$ and/or PR$^+$, HER2$^+$, and low Ki67 (<14%)
Luminal B	ER$^+$ and/or PR$^+$, HER2$^+$, and high Ki67 (≥14%)
	ER$^+$ and/or PR$^+$ and HER2$^+$ (luminal-HER2 group)
HER2	ER$^-$, PR$^-$, and HER2$^+$
Triple negative	ER$^-$, PR$^-$, HER2$^-$

Table 1.
Molecular profiles of different breast cancer subtypes.

2.2 Current treatment options for ER$^+$ breast cancer

2.2.1 Surgery

In general, surgery is the only way to cure most malignancies originated from solid organs. After diagnosis, patients with breast cancer in early stage should undertake surgery with or without radiotherapy, irrespective to the subtypes of breast cancer. There are two major surgical approaches for breast cancers—mastectomy (removal of the whole breast) and lumpectomy (breast-conserving therapy). The appealing advantage of lumpectomy enables patients to preserve their breast without compromising survival outcome. With the addition of radiotherapy following lumpectomy, survival outcomes have been reported to be equivalent to those after mastectomy as primary disease control in breast cancers with early stage [5–7].

Besides primary tumor resection, axillary lymph node (ALN) dissection or sentinel lymph node (SLN) biopsy and resection is also essentially performed on breast cancer patients to determine possible spread of cancer cells to lymph nodes from the original breast tumor. If the SLN examination reveals no evidence of malignant cell involvement, any other area of the body without cancer cell metastases would be highly postulated. Notably, the effectiveness of the SLN procedure to determine the presence of lymph node metastases is demonstrated to be identical to that of ALN dissection in various clinical studies.

2.2.2 Selective estrogen receptor modulators (SERMs)

The anti-breast cancer function of SERMs is mainly contributed by the competition with estrogen on ER, and modulations on ER-ERE (i.e. a type of gene promoter recognized by the activated ER) activity by altering the cooperated transcription factors in breast cancer cells (**Figure 1**) [8]. For both premenopausal and postmenopausal patients, the most commonly used SERM with established benefit in adjuvant setting is tamoxifen. Interestingly, although tamoxifen exhibits anti-estrogenic properties in the breast including the breast cancer cells; it exhibits estrogenic properties in bones and endometrial tissues. In ER$^+$ breast cancers, the use of tamoxifen after surgery could decrease the risk of recurrence as well as death [9–11].

In general, if both chemotherapy and hormone therapy are indicated for patients after surgery, the recommended sequence of management is initial chemotherapy following with the use of tamoxifen. Traditionally, tamoxifen is given to patients with early breast cancer for 5 years after primary surgery. In fact, the NCCN guidelines recommend patients to receive at least 5 years of treatment, if tamoxifen is considered to be used after surgery. However, results from the recent randomized Adjuvant Tamoxifen: Longer Against Shorter (ATLAS) study have supported 10 years of tamoxifen treatment in the adjuvant setting. The risks of disease recurrence and death were shown to be decreased in patients completing 10 years of tamoxifen treatment, as compared with those for 5 years of treatment, despite the increased risks of getting endometrial cancer and pulmonary embolism [9]. Based on these findings, adjuvant tamoxifen treatment for 10 years is now considered for patients with early breast cancer. The NCCN guidelines also recommend tamoxifen treatment for ER⁺ metastatic breast cancer patients.

Toremifene is another SERM which has demonstrated its clinical efficacy in ER⁺ breast cancers. Several studies have shown equivalent efficacy of toremifene in disease control of metastatic breast cancers, as compared with tamoxifen [12, 13]. Therefore, similar to tamoxifen, toremifene is also recommended in NCCN guidelines for disease control in patients with ER⁺ metastatic breast cancers.

2.2.3 Aromatase inhibitors (AIs)

Aromatase is an enzyme that belongs to the family of cytochrome P-450 and it is responsible for the conversion of androgens to estrogens in peripheral tissues. Given that this peripheral conversion by the aromatase is the main origin of estrogen production in postmenopausal women, inhibition of this particular enzyme could lead to the significant reduction of estrogens (**Figure 1**). AIs are now suggested to be the standard of care for postmenopausal patients with ER⁺ breast cancer in NCCN guidelines. Current AIs could be grouped into two different subtypes—steroidal and non-steroidal AIs. Steroidal AIs, also termed as type I inhibitors, have steroid-like structure similar to the substrate of aromatase. This similarity confers these AIs the ability to interact with the substrate-binding site of aromatase and subsequent inactivation of this enzyme. Non-steroidal AIs or type II inhibitors could bind to the heme moiety of the aromatase non-covalently, and therefore prevent binding of androgens. Unlike type I inhibitor, the inhibition of androgen by this type of AIs is reversible by competitive binding of androgens. There are currently one type I inhibitor (i.e. exemestane) and two type II inhibitors (i.e. letrozole and anastrozole) approved by the US Food and Drug Administration (FDA). They are all indicated in both the adjuvant and metastatic setting for postmenopausal patients with ER⁺ breast cancer (**Table 2**).

Several studies have been carried out to evaluate the effects of different therapeutic strategies of AIs in the treatment of postmenopausal patients with early stage ER⁺ breast cancer. Different therapeutic strategies including (1) initial treatment with AIs, (2) sequential therapy with AIs after 2–3 years of tamoxifen, and (3) extended therapy with AIs after the completion of tamoxifen for 5 years have been extensively studied. Two phase III pivotal studies, named ATAC [14] and BIG 1-98 [15], have demonstrated the clinical efficacy of 5 years of adjuvant AIs (i.e. initial treatment with AIs). However, the hazard ratio (HR) for disease-free survival (DFS) comparing 5 years of tamoxifen of these studies, ranging from 0.81 to 0.91, indicates minimal improvement of the use of AIs to prevent disease recurrence after surgery. Several clinical studies, such as ARNO 95 [16], ITA [17], and IES [18] have shown the clinical benefit of sequential treatment of AI after 2–3 years of tamoxifen. In patients receiving sequential therapy comparing with 5 years of tamoxifen, HR for DFS ranges from 0.57 to 0.76. In extended therapy of AIs beyond 5 years of tamoxifen, its clinical efficacy in the reduction of HR for DFS, ranging from 0.58 to 0.68, has also been reported in randomized studies [19, 20]. According to the NCCN guidelines, the abovementioned AIs related strategies (i.e. AIs as initial adjuvant therapy for 5 years; 2–3 years of tamoxifen followed by AIs to complete 5 years of adjuvant therapy; and 5 years of tamoxifen followed by 5 years of AIs) are all recommended for postmenopausal breast cancer patients who are required for receiving adjuvant hormone therapy.

Trial	Disease setting	Study group	Control group	Significant findings
ATAC [14]	Adjuvant	Anastrozole for 5 years	Tamoxifen for 5 years	HR for DFS: 0.91
BIG1-98 [15]	Adjuvant	Letrozole for 5 years	Tamoxifen for 5 years	HR for DFS: 0.81
ARNO95 [16]	Adjuvant	2 years of tamoxifen +3 years of anastrozole	Tamoxifen for 5 years	HR for DFS: 0.66
ITA [17]	Adjuvant	2–3 years of tamoxifen followed by anastrozole to complete total 5 years of HT	Tamoxifen for 5 years	HR for DFS: 0.56
IES [18]	Adjuvant	2–3 years of tamoxifen followed by exemestane to complete total 5 years of HT	Tamoxifen for 5 years	HR for DFS: 0.76
MA17 [19]	Adjuvant	4.5–6 years of tamoxifen +5 years of letrozole	Tamoxifen for 5 years	HR for DFS: 0.58
B33 [20]	Adjuvant	5 years of tamoxifen +5 years of exemestane	Tamoxifen for 5 years	HR for DFS: 0.68

DFS, disease-free survival; HT, hormone therapy; HR, hazard ratio.

Table 2.
Clinical benefits of using aromatase inhibitors in ER⁺ breast cancers.

In metastatic disease, improved survival outcomes of applying AIs as the first-line hormone therapy as compared with using tamoxifen in postmenopausal patients have also been revealed in studies conducted by Arimidex Study Group, International Letrozole Breast Cancer Group, and the EORTC Breast Group [21–23]. Although this advantage is small, AIs are still recommended by NCCN for use in treating ER⁺ metastatic breast cancer in postmenopausal patients.

2.2.4 Selective estrogen receptor degrader (SERD)

Unlike SERMs that function as partial competitive antagonists of ER, SERDs are antiestrogens designed to destabilize ER of tumor cells (**Figure 1**). After binding to ERs, SERDs could induce the degradation of these receptors, and thereby lead to the inhibition of estrogen associated signaling pathway [24]. Fulvestrant is the only SERD approved by FDA for clinical use in the management of ER⁺ breast cancers. Equivalent effect of fulvestrant on tumor response rate and time to progression, as compared with AIs, have been reported in postmenopausal patients with progressive metastatic ER⁺ breast cancer following prior hormone therapy [25, 26]. In NCCN guidelines, fulvestrant is suggested in clinical use of postmenopausal metastatic ER⁺ breast cancers.

2.2.5 Luteinizing hormone-releasing hormone (LHRH) analogs

Ovary is the major organ responsible for estrogen production. Therefore, oophorectomy has been recognized as one of the effective treatments for premenopausal patients with metastatic ER⁺ breast cancers. Besides oophorectomy, medical treatments with LHRH analogs have also been used clinically to ablate ovary function for over 30 years [27]. Through desensitizing gonadotropin-releasing hormone (GnRH) receptors, LHRH analogs suppress the secretion of gonadotropin, luteinizing hormone (LH) and follicle-stimulating hormone (FSH), resulting in reduced estrogen levels in the body (**Figure 1**). Although a combination of LHRH analogs and SERMs has been demonstrated to improve survivals significantly as compared to chemo-therapy alone [28], further studies indicate that in premenopausal patients with ER$^+$ early breast cancer, adjuvant treatment with LHRH analogs combined with SERMs (tamoxifen) does not carry any clinical benefits [29]. However, the combination of LHRH analogs and AIs (i.e. exemestane) as an adjuvant therapy significantly reduces the risk of recurrence in premenopausal patients with early disease [30]. In metastatic diseases, both the combinations of LHRH analogs and SERMs or AIs have shown the benefit of survivals in premenopausal patients [31–33]. In NCCN guidelines, LHRH analogs are recommended to use in combination with AIs or SERMs in premeno-pausal patients with ER$^+$ breast cancer, both in adjuvant or metastatic setting.

2.3. Mechanisms of hormone therapy resistance in ER$^+$ breast cancer

Despite various hormone therapy agents have been developed and proven to be effective in treating ER$^+$ early stage breast cancer, intrinsic and acquired resistance to hormone therapy are frequently observed in breast cancer patients. In the follow-ing sections, we will discuss the biology behind the induction of hormone therapy resistance in ER$^+$ breast cancer in details.

2.3.1 Dysregulation and conformation alteration of ERα

Under normal physiological conditions, the binding of estrogen to ER will trigger ER conformation changes and ER dimerization (e.g. ERαβ heterodimer formations). Then, the activated ER dimers will bind onto the estrogen response elements (EREs; promotor regions specifically recognized by the activated ER dimers) and drive the expression of the ERE-regulated cell survival- and growth-related genes. Decreased ERα expression (and aberrant ERα protein conformation) and reduced survival dependence on the estrogen-ER signaling pathway are both known to promote hormone therapy resistance in ER$^+$ breast cancer. For example, upregulation of the zinc-finger-homeodomain transcription factor, zinc-finger E-box binding homeobox 1 (ZEB1), has been shown to downregulate ERα expression epigenetically through formation of a ZEB1/DNA methyltransferase 3B (DNMT3B)/histone deacetylase 1 (HDAC1) complex on the promoter of ERα and to induce tamoxifen resistance in breast cancer cells. High ZEB1 expressions also correlate with ERα promoter hyper-methylation and reduced ERα expression in breast cancer patients [34].

As described in the above sections, tamoxifen is a SERM that exhibits differential effects on ER conformation and ER-signaling pathways. Despite tamoxifen inhibits the ER-ERE-related survival-signaling pathways in ER$^+$ breast cancer cells and this drug is widely used to treat ER$^+$ breast cancer; tamoxifen is known to increase the risk of having endometrial proliferation, endometrial hyperplasia, endometrial cancer, and uterine sarcomas in the treated breast cancer patients, possibly through activation of the ER-signaling pathways in endometrial cells. Phosphorylation of the amino acid residue serine-305 in the hinge region of ERα by protein kinase A (PKA) has been demonstrated to change the resulting conformation of ERα upon tamoxifen interactions, turning the tamoxifen-bound ERα from an inactive form into an active form (i.e. tamoxifen acts as an ER-agonist), leading to the activation of ER-ERE signaling pathways in ER$^+$ breast cancer cells (**Figure 2**) [35].

2.3.2 Dysregulation of cell survival-related signaling pathways and pro-/anti-apoptotic molecules

It is widely demonstrated that aberrant downregulation of p53, upregulation of human epidermal growth factor receptor 2 (HER2/neu), the phosphatidylinositol

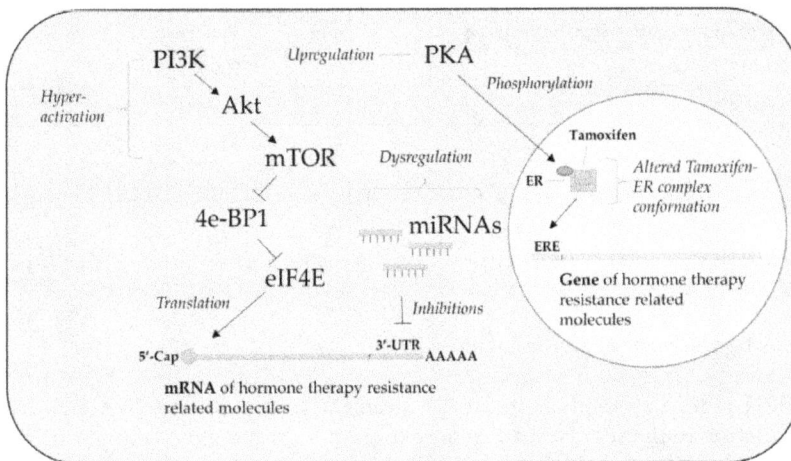

Figure 2.
Picture showing a few molecules and molecular pathways that are involved in the induction of hormone therapy resistance in ER⁺ breast cancer cells.

3-kinase/protein kinase B/mammalian target of rapamycin [PI3K/PKB(Akt)/mTOR]-signaling pathway, and the extracellular signal-regulated kinases (ERK, also called MAPK)-signaling pathway can promote the survival and metastasis of cancer cells. In fact, dysregulation of these molecules and signaling pathways has also been found in the ER⁺ hormone therapy resistance breast cancer cells (**Figure 2**). For example, a study by Liang et al. revealed that melanoma cell adhesion molecule (MCAM, also called CD146 or MUC18) negatively regulates ERα expression, but positively regulates the Akt-signaling pathway, in breast cancer cells. Moreover, increased expression of MCAM was found to induce epithelial-mesenchymal transition (EMT) and tamoxifen resistance *via* Akt-signaling pathway activation in the tamoxifen-resistance breast cancer cells in the same study [36].

Survivin is a well-known anti-apoptotic and pro-tumorigenic molecule. It contains a single baculovirus inhibitor of apoptosis protein repeat (BIR) domain and it is believed that survivin binds to caspases through its BIR domain and subsequently inhibits the activity of caspases. On the other hand, survivin forms chromosomal passenger complex (CPC) with aurora B kinase, borealin, and inner centromere protein (INCENP) and successful formation of CPC plays an important role in chromosome segregation during mitosis [37, 38]. Survivin protein translation is known to be positively regulated by the Akt/mTOR-signaling pathway and dysregulation of the Akt/mTOR/survivin pathway is known to be a factor of estrogen-independence and tamoxifen-resistance causation in the MCF7-derived ER⁺ breast cancer cells [39]. Of note, hyper-phosphorylation of the survivin-binding partner, aurora B kinase, has also been demonstrated to be capable of causing fulvestrant resistance in ER⁺ T47D breast cancer cells [40].

Besides dysregulation of the Akt/mTOR-signaling pathway, Yin et al. revealed that upregulation of G protein-coupled estrogen receptor (GPER) triggers Erk-signaling pathway activation, leading to the expression reduction of the BH3-only pro-apoptotic molecule, Bim, and induction of tamoxifen resistance in ER⁺ breast cancer [41]. Myeloid cell leukemia-1 (Mcl-1) is a suppressor of Bim and overexpression of this anti-apoptotic molecule has also been found in MCF7-derived antiestrogen-resistant cancer cell lines [42]. Other molecules/pathways that have been found to play a role in the induction of hormone therapy resistance in ER⁺ breast cancer are listed in **Table 3**.

Name of the molecule or signaling pathway	Reference
MTDH-PTEN-Akt	Xu et al. [43]
Plk1-Cdc25c	Jeong et al. [44]
RUNX2-ER-SOX9	Jeselsohn et al. [45]
Rac1-PAK1	Gonzalez et al. [46]

Table 3.
List of molecules/pathways known to contribute to the induction of hormone therapy resistance in ER⁺ breast cancer during dysregulated situations.

2.3.3 Dysregulation of microRNAs (miRNAs)

MiRNAs are a class of small (20–22 nucleotides) non-coding RNA molecules that function in the regulation of gene expression. At the molecular level, miRNAs bind onto mRNAs at specific locations (putative binding sites) through complementary base-pairing and subsequently inhibit the translation of the targeted genes. Given that the expression of various tumor suppressors and oncoproteins is known to be regulated by miRNAs; dysregulation of miRNAs is believed as one of the causes of tumorigenesis, tumor metastasis, and tumor drug resistance in human.

Aberrant expression of different miRNAs has been shown to contribute to the induction of hormone therapy resistance through downstream modulations of different cell survival or division-related signaling molecules in ER⁺ breast cancer (**Figure 2**). For example, we found in a previous study that the MCF7-derived, ER⁺ hormone therapy-resistant (i.e. estrogen independent and tamoxifen resistant) breast cancer cells, which were generated in our laboratory, exhibits reduced expression of miR-125a-5p but increased expression of survivin as compared to the parental hormone therapy sensitive MCF7 cells. We also found that miR-125a-5p is an expression suppressor of survivin and dysregulation of the HDAC2/5-miR-125a-5p-survivin pathway in part contributes to the induction of estrogen independence and tamoxifen resistance in the same breast cancer cell line [39]. The role of miR-125a-5p downregulation in hormone therapy resistance induction is further supported by clinical data analysis showing that low miR-125a-5p expression levels correlate with poor overall survival in tamoxifen-treated ER⁺ breast cancer patients [39]. Induction of tamoxifen resistance has also been shown in ER⁺ breast cancer cells with dysregulation of miR-125a-3p, a molecule which is closely related to miR-125a-5p. A study by Zheng et al. revealed that miR-125a-3p is an inhibitor of cyclin-dependent kinase 3 (cdk3), which is an ER transcriptional activity enhancer, in ER⁺ breast cancer cells. In addition, reduced expression of miR-125a-3p and increased expression of cdk3 was found in the ER⁺ tamoxifen-resistant breast cancer cells and ectopic overexpression of miR-125a-3p was shown to decrease the expression of cdk3 and restore the sensitivity to tamoxifen in the same cell line *in vitro* [47].

Metabolic reprogramming is believed as one of the mechanisms that can promote drug resistance in cancer cells. Interestingly, aberrant upregulation of miR-155 has been found to drive metabolic reprogramming *via* miR-143 downregulation and hexokinase-2 (HK2; a glycolysis-priming enzyme and a known target of miR-143) upregulation, promoting the survival of ER⁺ breast cancer cells under estrogen-deprived conditions (mimics aromatase inhibitors treatment) [48]. Other miRNAs that have been found to play a role in the induction of hormone therapy resistance in ER⁺ breast cancer are listed in **Table 4**.

Name of microRNA	Demonstrated effects in ER⁺ breast cancer cells	Reference
miR-27b	Tamoxifen resistant	Li et al. [49]
miR-214	Fulvestrant resistant Tamoxifen resistant	Yu et al. [50]
miR-320a	Tamoxifen resistant	Lü et al. [51]
miR-375	Tamoxifen resistant	Ward et al. [52]
miR-378a-3p	Estrogen independent (*aromatase inhibitors-resistant*) Tamoxifen resistant	Ikeda et al. [53]

Table 4.
List of miRNAs known to contribute to the induction of hormone therapy resistance in ER⁺ breast cancer during dysregulated situations.

2.3.4 Tumor microenvironment

Emerging evidences suggest that altered tumor microenvironment promotes drug resistance induction and malignant progression of cancer. As a tumor grows, tumor cells located at a distal distance from blood vessels will experience a hypoxic environment and eventually some of the severe hypoxia-experienced tumor cell will undergo necrosis or apoptosis. However, tumor cells are known to be capable of carrying a series of cellular and molecular changes in order to maintain their survival and also to promote tumor progression under hypoxic conditions. For example, it has been reported that hypoxia induces downregulation of ERα, upregulation of hypoxia-inducible factor 1α (HIF-1α; a transcription factor known promote the expression of various cell survival-related proteins) and vascular endothelial growth factor (VEGF; a growth factor known to promote angiogenesis) expressions, and promotes the development of estrogen independence in ER⁺ breast cancer cells *in vitro*.

Cancer-associated fibroblasts (CAFs) have been implicated in the development of hormone therapy resistance in ER⁺ breast cancer [54, 55]. It has been demonstrated that CD146-negative CAFs suppress ER expression in ER⁺ breast cancer cells, decrease tumor cell sensitivity to estrogen, and increase tumor cell resistance to tamoxifen therapy [55]. As mentioned in the previous section, GPER upregulation triggers Erk-signaling pathway activation and Bim downregulation in ER⁺ breast cancer cells. A study by Yuan et al. demonstrated that GPER also positively regulates the expression of an adhesion molecule, β1-integrin, and the downstream molecules of β1-integrin, FAK, and Scr, in the MCF7-derived tamoxifen-resistant breast cancer cells. Importantly, they further showed that the product of CAFs, fibronectin, interacts with β1-integrin and promotes epithelial-mesenchymal transition (EMT) in breast cancer cells [56].

3. Combating ER⁺ hormone therapy-resistant breast cancer

As described in the above sections, overexpression of survivin, aurora B kinase, and Mcl-1 has been found in different ER⁺ hormone therapy-resistant breast cancer models. In fact, survivin, aurora B kinase, and Mcl-1 are all known to play important roles in maintaining cancer cells survival and metastasis in ER⁺ breast cancer, HER2⁺ breast cancer, and the triple-negative breast cancer. Therefore, it is not surprising to see that the effectiveness of a group of survivin, aurora B kinase, and Mcl-1 inhibitors in targeting ER⁺ hormone therapy-resistant breast cancer has been investigated extensively in different pre-clinical studies. For example, a small molecule inhibitor of survivin, YM155 (sepantronium bromide), has previously been demonstrated to exhibit similar potency in MCF7 and MCF7-derived ER$^+$ tamoxifen-resistant breast cancer cells regardless to the expression of p53 [57]. Interestingly, the 3-hydroxy-3-methylglutaryl coenzyme A (HMG-CoA) reductase inhibitor and the anti-cholesteremic agent, lovastatin (mevacor), has been shown to decrease survivin expression and increase the therapeutic effect of tamoxifen in tamoxifen-resistant breast cancer cells [58]. Targeting aurora B kinase by small molecule inhibitor, AZD1152 (barasertib), has also been shown to potentiate the effects of fulvestrant in patient-derived estrogen-independent ER$^+$ breast cancer cells [40]. Moreover, a dual aurora kinase and cyclin-dependent kinase inhibitor, JNJ-7706621, and a deubiquitinase inhibitor (i.e. capable of destabilizing Mcl-1), WP1130, have both been demonstrated to be functional in promoting the death of tamoxifen-resistant breast cancer cells [42].

SAHA (vorinostat) is an epigenetic modulator [histone deacetylase inhibitor (HDACi)] that was approved by the US FDA for the treatment of cutaneous T cell lymphoma on 2006. A study by Lee et al. revealed that SAHA preferentially inhibits HDAC3, HDAC6 and their downstream targets, survivin and XIAP, in MCF7 and MDA-MB-231 breast cancer cells *in vitro* [59]. Notably, a phase II clinical study revealed that the combination of SAHA and tamoxifen exhibited encouraging activity in reversing hormone resistance in patients with hormone therapy-resistant breast cancer [60]. Besides epigenetic modulators, the possibility of using Akt/ mTOR-signaling pathway inhibitors in treating ER$^+$ hormone therapy-resistant breast cancer has also been evaluated in different pre-clinical and clinical studies. For example, the orally bioavailable ATP-competitive mTOR inhibitor, AZD8055, was found to be more potent against the proliferation of the MCF7-derived tamoxifen-resistant breast cancer cells than that of parent cells [61]. In addition, co-treatment with the mTOR inhibitor, rapamycin (sirolimus), was shown to be capable of restoring tamoxifen sensitivity in ER$^+$ tamoxifen-resistant breast cancer cells [62]. AZD5363 is a pan-Akt kinase catalytic inhibitor and it is currently in phase I clinical trials for various cancers. A study by Ribas et al. demonstrated that AZD5363 was capable of inhibiting the growth of the ER$^+$ estrogen-independent MCF7-LTED, T47D-LTED, and ZR75-LTED breast cancer cells at the low-to-middle nanomolar range *in vitro*. In addition, combination of AZD5363 with fulvestrant was shown to exhibit synergistic anticancer effects in a patient-derived luminal breast cancer xenograft HBCx22OvaR model [63]. The pan-class I PI3K inhibitor, BKM120 (buparlisib), is currently in a phase III study in combination with fulvestrant in postmenopausal patients with ER$^+$, HER2$^-$ breast cancer refractory to non-steroidal aromatase inhibitors (ClinicalTrials.gov Identifier: NCT01610284).

4. Conclusion

Since hormone therapy is the mainstay of treatment in early ER$^+$ breast cancer, hormone therapy resistance represents the major challenge in the management of this disease. Dysregulation of various cell survival-signaling pathways (such as Akt/ mTOR and PI3K) and molecules (like HDACs, survivin, and miR-125a-5p) in breast cancer cells and CAFs in tumor microenvironment is now known to contribute to the induction of hormone therapy resistance in ER$^+$ breast cancer. Therefore, co-treatments of mTOR inhibitors like rapamycin or HDACi like SAHA with SERMs/ AIs may give better therapeutic (i.e. clinical) outcomes in patients with advanced/ hormone therapy-resistant ER$^+$ breast cancer in the future. Furthermore, even though the effectiveness of hormone therapy in patients with ER$^+$ breast cancer can be predicted based on their breast cancer subtypes classified according to the results of the pre-treatment pathological examinations using IHC and PAM50 (Prosigna®); however, there is still room for the improvement of the current breast cancer pathological classification system as intrinsic resistance to hormone therapy is frequently found in patients with breast cancer predicted to be hormone therapy sensitive. A better breast cancer pathological classification system is needed for the development of personalized breast cancer treatments in the future.

Acknowledgements

Publication of this chapter is supported by the Ministry of Science and Technology and National Cheng Kung University of Taiwan.

Conflict of interest

Authors declared no conflict of interest.

Author details

Shang-Hung Chen[1,2†] and Chun Hei Antonio Cheung[3,4*†]

1 National Institute of Cancer Research, National Health Research Institutes, Tainan, Taiwan

2 Division of Hematology and Oncology, Department of Internal Medicine, National Cheng Kung University Hospital, College of Medicine, National Cheng Kung University, Tainan, Taiwan

3 Department of Pharmacology, College of Medicine, National Cheng Kung University, Tainan, Taiwan

4 Institute of Basic Medical Sciences, College of Medicine, National Cheng Kung University, Tainan, Taiwan

*Address all correspondence to: acheung@mail.ncku.edu.tw

†These authors contributed equally.

IntechOpen

References

[1] Pestalozzi BC et al. Distinct clinical and prognostic features of infiltrating lobular carcinoma of the breast: Combined results of 15 International Breast Cancer Study Group clinical trials. Journal of Clinical Oncology. 2008;**26**(18):3006-3014

[2] Spitale A et al. Breast cancer classification according to immunohistochemical markers: Clinicopathologic features and short-term survival analysis in a population-based study from the south of Switzerland. Annals of Oncology. 2009;**20**(4):628-635

[3] Vallejos CS et al. Breast cancer classification according to immunohistochemistry markers: Subtypes and association with clinicopathologic variables in a Peruvian hospital database. Clinical Breast Cancer. 2010;**10**(4):294-300

[4] Goldhirsch A et al. Thresholds for therapies: Highlights of the St Gallen International Expert Consensus on the primary therapy of early breast cancer 2009. Annals of Oncology. 2009;**20**(8):1319-1329

[5] Arriagada R et al. Conservative treatment versus mastectomy in early breast cancer: Patterns of failure with 15 years of follow-up data. Institut Gustave-Roussy Breast Cancer Group. Journal of Clinical Oncology. 1996;**14**(5):1558-1564

[6] Fisher B et al. Twenty-year follow-up of a randomized trial comparing total mastectomy, lumpectomy, and lumpectomy plus irradiation for the treatment of invasive breast cancer. The New England Journal of Medicine. 2002;**347**(16):1233-1241

[7] Clarke M et al. Effects of radiotherapy and of differences in the extent of surgery for early breast cancer on local recurrence and 15-year survival: An overview of the randomised trials. Lancet. 2005;**366**(9503):2087-2106

[8] Nilsson S, Koehler KF. Oestrogen receptors and selective oestrogen receptor modulators: Molecular and cellular pharmacology. Basic & Clinical Pharmacology & Toxicology. 2005;**96**(1):15-25

[9] Davies C et al. Long-term effects of continuing adjuvant tamoxifen to 10 years versus stopping at 5 years after diagnosis of oestrogen receptor-positive breast cancer: ATLAS, a randomised trial. The Lancet. 2013;**381**(9869):805-816

[10] Albain KS et al. Adjuvant chemotherapy and timing of tamoxifen in postmenopausal patients with endocrine-responsive, node-positive breast cancer: A phase 3, open-label, randomised controlled trial. Lancet. 2009;**374**(9707):2055-2063

[11] Early Breast Cancer Trialists' Collaborative G, et al. Relevance of breast cancer hormone receptors and other factors to the efficacy of adjuvant tamoxifen: Patient-level meta-analysis of randomised trials. Lancet. 2011;**378**(9793):771-784

[12] Pyrhönen S et al. Comparison of toremifene and tamoxifen in post-menopausal patients with advanced breast cancer: A randomized double-blind, the 'nordic' phase III study. British Journal of Cancer. 1997;**76**:270

[13] Milla-Santos A et al. Phase III randomized trial of toremifene vs tamoxifen in hormonodependant advanced breast cancer. Breast Cancer Research and Treatment. 2001;**65**(2):119-124

[14] Arimidex Tamoxifen Alone or in Combination (ATAC) Trialists' Group, et al. Effect of anastrozole and tamoxifen as adjuvant treatment for early-stage breast cancer: 100-month analysis of the ATAC trial. The Lancet Oncology. 2008;**9**(1):45-53

[15] B I G Collaborative Group, et al. Letrozole therapy alone or in sequence with tamoxifen in women with breast cancer. New England Journal of Medicine. 2009;**361**(8):766-776

[16] Kaufmann M et al. Improved overall survival in postmenopausal women with early breast cancer after anastrozole initiated after treatment with Tamoxifen compared with continued tamoxifen: The ARNO 95 study. Journal of Clinical Oncology. 2007;**25**(19):2664-2670

[17] Boccardo F et al. Switching to anastrozole versus continued tamoxifen treatment of early breast cancer. Updated results of the Italian tamoxifen anastrozole (ITA) trial. Annals of Oncology. 2006;**17**(Suppl 7):vii10-vii14

[18] Coombes RC et al. Survival and safety of exemestane versus tamoxifen after 2-3 years' tamoxifen treatment (Intergroup Exemestane Study): A randomised controlled trial. Lancet. 2007;**369**(9561):559-570

[19] Goss PE et al. Efficacy of letrozole extended adjuvant therapy according to estrogen receptor and progesterone receptor status of the primary tumor: National Cancer Institute of Canada Clinical Trials Group MA.17. Journal of Clinical Oncology. 2007;**25**(15):2006-2011

[20] Mamounas EP et al. Benefit from exemestane as extended adjuvant therapy after 5 years of adjuvant tamoxifen: Intention-to-treat analysis of the National Surgical Adjuvant Breast and Bowel Project B-33

Trial. Journal of Clinical Oncology. 2008;**26**(12):1965-1971

[21] Nabholtz JM et al. Anastrozole is superior to tamoxifen as first-line therapy for advanced breast cancer in postmenopausal women: Results of a North American Multicenter Randomized trial. Journal of Clinical Oncology. 2000;**18**(22):3758-3767

[22] Mouridsen H et al. Phase III study of Letrozole versus tamoxifen as first-line therapy of advanced breast cancer in postmenopausal women: Analysis of survival and update of efficacy from the international letrozole breast cancer group. Journal of Clinical Oncology. 2003;**21**(11):2101-2109

[23] Paridaens R, et al. First line hormonal treatment (HT) for metastatic breast cancer (MBC) with exemestane (E) or tamoxifen (T) in postmenopausal patients (pts)—A randomized phase III trial of the EORTC Breast Group. Journal of Clinical Oncology. 2004;**22**(14_suppl):515

[24] McDonnell DP, Wardell SE. The molecular mechanisms underlying the pharmacological actions of ER modulators: Implications for new drug discovery in breast cancer. Current Opinion in Pharmacology. 2010;**10**(6):620-628

[25] Ellis MJ et al. Fulvestrant 500 mg versus anastrozole 1 mg for the FIRST-line treatment of advanced breast cancer: Overall survival analysis from the phase II FIRST study. Journal of Clinical Oncology. 2015;**33**(32):3781-3787

[26] Chia S et al. Double-blind, randomized placebo controlled trial of fulvestrant compared with exemestane after prior nonsteroidal aromatase inhibitor therapy in postmenopausal women with hormone receptor–positive, advanced breast cancer:

Results from EFECT. Journal of Clinical Oncology. 2008;**26**(10):1664-1670

[27] Nourmoussavi M et al. Ovarian ablation for premenopausal breast cancer: A review of treatment considerations and the impact of premature menopause. Cancer Treatment Reviews. 2017;**55**:26-35

[28] Davidson NE et al. Chemoendocrine therapy for premenopausal women with axillary lymph node–positive, steroid hormone receptor–positive breast cancer: Results from INT 0101 (E5188). Journal of Clinical Oncology. 2005;**23**(25):5973-5982

[29] LHRH-agonists in Early Breast Cancer Overview group. Use of luteinising-hormone-releasing hormone agonists as adjuvant treatment in premenopausal patients with hormone-receptor-positive breast cancer: A meta-analysis of individual patient data from randomised adjuvant trials. The Lancet. 2007;**369**(9574):1711-1723

[30] Pagani O et al. Adjuvant exemestane with ovarian suppression in premenopausal breast cancer. The New England Journal of Medicine. 2014;**371**(2):107-118

[31] Jonat W et al. A randomised study to compare the effect of the luteinising hormone releasing hormone (LHRH) analogue goserelin with or without tamoxifen in pre- and perimenopausal patients with advanced breast cancer. European Journal of Cancer. 1995;**31**(2):137-142

[32] Carlson RW et al. Phase II trial of anastrozole plus goserelin in the treatment of hormone receptor-positive, metastatic carcinoma of the breast in premenopausal women. Journal of Clinical Oncology. 2010;**28**(25):3917-3921

[33] Yao S et al. Goserelin plus letrozole as first- or second-line hormonal treatment in premenopausal patients with advanced breast cancer. Endocrine Journal. 2011;**58**(6):509-516

[34] Zhang JB et al. ZEB1 induces ER-alpha promoter hypermethylation and confers antiestrogen resistance in breast cancer. Cell Death & Disease. 2017;**8**:e2732

[35] Michalides R et al. Tamoxifen resistance by a conformational arrest of the estrogen receptor alpha after PKA activation in breast cancer. Cancer Cell. 2004;**5**(6):597-605

[36] Liang YK et al. MCAM/CD146 promotes tamoxifen resistance in breast cancer cells through induction of epithelial-mesenchymal transition, decreased ERalpha expression and AKT activation. Cancer Letters. 2017;**386**:65-76

[37] Vader G et al. Survivin mediates targeting of the chromosomal passenger complex to the centromere and midbody. EMBO Reports. 2006;**7**(1):85-92

[38] Jeyaprakash AA et al. Structure of a survivin-borealin-INCENP core complex reveals how chromosomal passengers travel together. Cell. 2007;**131**(2):271-285

[39] Huang WT et al. HDAC2 and HDAC5 up-regulations modulate survivin and miR-125a-5p expressions and promote hormone therapy resistance in estrogen receptor positive breast cancer cells. Frontiers in Pharmacology. 2017;**8**:902

[40] Larsen SL et al. Aurora kinase B is important for antiestrogen resistant cell growth and a potential biomarker for tamoxifen resistant breast cancer. BMC Cancer. 2015;**15**(1):239

[41] Yin H et al. GPER promotes tamoxifen-resistance in ER+ breast cancer cells by reduced Bim proteins

through MAPK/Erk-TRIM2 signaling axis. International Journal of Oncology. 2017;**51**(4):1191-1198

[42] Thrane S et al. A kinase inhibitor screen identifies Mcl-1 and aurora kinase a as novel treatment targets in antiestrogen-resistant breast cancer cells. Oncogene. 2014;**34**:4199

[43] Xu CY et al. MTDH mediates estrogen-independent growth and tamoxifen resistance by down-regulating PTEN in MCF-7 breast cancer cells. Cellular Physiology and Biochemistry. 2014;**33**(5):1557-1567

[44] Jeong SB et al. Essential role of polo-like kinase 1 (Plk1) oncogene in tumor growth and metastasis of tamoxifen-resistant breast cancer. Molecular Cancer Therapeutics. 2018;**17**(4):825-837

[45] Jeselsohn R et al. Embryonic transcription factor SOX9 drives breast cancer endocrine resistance. Proceedings of the National Academy of Sciences of the United States of America. 2017;**114**(22):E4482-E4491

[46] Gonzalez N et al. Pharmacological inhibition of Rac1-PAK1 axis restores tamoxifen sensitivity in human resistant breast cancer cells. Cellular Signalling. 2017;**30**:154-161

[47] Zheng L et al. miR-125a-3p inhibits ERalpha transactivation and overrides tamoxifen resistance by targeting CDK3 in estrogen receptor-positive breast cancer. The FASEB Journal. 2018;**32**(2):588-600

[48] Bacci M et al. miR-155 drives metabolic reprogramming of ER+ breast cancer cells following long-term estrogen deprivation and predicts clinical response to aromatase inhibitors. Cancer Research. 2016;**76**(6):1615-1626

[49] Li XN et al. MiR-27b is epigenetically downregulated in tamoxifen resistant breast cancer cells due to promoter methylation and regulates tamoxifen sensitivity by targeting HMGB3. Biochemical and Biophysical Research Communications. 2016;**477**(4):768-773

[50] Yu X et al. MiR-214 increases the sensitivity of breast cancer cells to tamoxifen and fulvestrant through inhibition of autophagy. Molecular Cancer. 2015;**14**:208

[51] Lu M et al. MicroRNA-320a sensitizes tamoxifen-resistant breast cancer cells to tamoxifen by targeting ARPP-19 and ERRgamma. Scientific Reports. 2015;**5**:8735

[52] Ward A et al. Re-expression of microRNA-375 reverses both tamoxifen resistance and accompanying EMT-like properties in breast cancer. Oncogene. 2013;**32**(9):1173-1182

[53] Ikeda K et al. miR-378a-3p modulates tamoxifen sensitivity in breast cancer MCF-7 cells through targeting GOLT1A. Scientific Reports. 2015;**5**:13170

[54] Shekhar MPV et al. Direct involvement of breast tumor fibroblasts in the modulation of tamoxifen sensitivity. The American Journal of Pathology. 2007;**170**(5):1546-1560

[55] Brechbuhl HM et al. Fibroblast subtypes regulate responsiveness of luminal breast cancer to estrogen. Clinical Cancer Research. 2017;**23**(7):1710

[56] Yuan J et al. Acquisition of epithelial-mesenchymal transition phenotype in the tamoxifen-resistant breast cancer cell: A new role for G protein-coupled estrogen receptor in mediating tamoxifen resistance through cancer-associated fibroblast-derived fibronectin and beta1-integrin signaling pathway in tumor cells. Breast Cancer Research. 2015;**17**:69

[57] Cheng SM et al. YM155 down-regulates survivin and XIAP, modulates autophagy and induces autophagy-dependent DNA damage in breast cancer cells. British Journal of Pharmacology. 2015;**172**(1):214-234

[58] Moriai R et al. Survivin plays as a resistant factor against tamoxifen-induced apoptosis in human breast cancer cells. Breast Cancer Research and Treatment. 2009;**117**:261-271

[59] Lee JY et al. Inhibition of HDAC3- and HDAC6-promoted survivin expression plays an important role in SAHA-induced autophagy and viability reduction in breast cancer cells. Frontiers in Pharmacology. 2016;7:81

[60] Munster PN et al. A phase II study of the histone deacetylase inhibitor vorinostat combined with tamoxifen for the treatment of patients with hormone therapy-resistant breast cancer. British Journal of Cancer. 2011;**104**(12):1828-1835

[61] Shi J-j et al. The mTOR inhibitor AZD8055 overcomes tamoxifen resistance in breast cancer cells by down-regulating HSPB8. Acta Pharmacologica Sinica. 2018; In Press

[62] deGraffenried LA et al. Inhibition of mTOR activity restores tamoxifen response in breast cancer cells with aberrant Akt activity. Clinical Cancer Research. 2004;**10**(23):8059

[63] Ribas R et al. AKT antagonist AZD5363 influences estrogen receptor function in endocrine-resistant breast cancer and synergizes with fulvestrant (ICI182780) in vivo. Molecular Cancer Therapeutics. 2015;**14**(9):2035-2048

Chapter 2

The Role of Metabolism in the Estrogenic Activity of Endocrine-Disrupting Chemicals

Darja Gramec Skledar and Lucija Peterlin Mašič

Abstract

Exposure to several natural and synthetic chemicals can disrupt the endocrine system and thus present a threat to human health. *In vivo*, such chemicals can be metabolized, which can change the endocrine activity of the parent chemical. Metabolism is usually considered to be a detoxification process, as it generally appears to reduce the estrogenic activity of a chemical and accelerate its elimination from the body. This is seen for bisphenol A (BPA), a known agonist of the estrogen receptor, whereby BPA glucuronide has no effects on this receptor. In contrast, numerous metabolites that show significantly greater estrogenic activities from their parent chemicals have been described in the literature. An example is the *ipso* metabolite of BPA, 4-methyl-2,4-bis(p-hydroxyphenyl)pent-1-ene, which shows >100-fold estrogenic activity compared to BPA. Consideration of metabolic pathways in *in vitro* models is therefore of great importance for reliable analysis and correct *in vitro* to *in vivo* correlations. The inclusion of metabolic aspects in these assays will reduce false-positive data for chemicals that are detoxified *in vivo* and false-negative data for proestrogens. Different approaches for this incorporation of metabolic systems for determination of estrogenic activities are already in use and are described in the present chapter.

Keywords: endocrine-disrupting chemicals, metabolic bioactivation, bisphenols, estrogenic activity, *in vitro* assays

1. Introduction

According to the World Health Organization definition from 2002, an endocrine-disrupting chemical (EDC) is an exogenous substance, or a mixture of substances, that alters the function(s) of the endocrine system and consequently that causes adverse health effects in the intact organism or its progeny or in (sub) populations [1]. The occurrence of EDCs in the environment is widespread, and exposure to EDCs is connected with many modern illnesses, such as cancers and metabolic syndrome [2, 3]. Effects of some EDCs on nuclear receptors have been reported even at very low doses, and thus EDCs have promoted increased concern among scientists and regulators [4–6]. As a result, over the last two decades, numerous *in vitro* and *in vivo* assays have been developed for the identification of EDCs [7, 8]. *In vitro* assays represent an important step, especially in the early stages of testing, as they can provide valuable information about the mechanisms of endocrine disruption (e.g., binding to the estrogen receptor [ER]). The main drawback of commonly used *in vitro* systems for estrogenic activity is that they do not consider pharmacokinetic parameters and especially the metabolism of a tested chemical [9].

Metabolism is the enzymatic process by which lipophilic compounds are transformed into hydrophilic metabolites, which can then be rapidly excreted with the urine. The liver is the main site of drug metabolism, although metabolic reactions also occur in extrahepatic tissues, like the gut and the airways [10]. Phase I metabolic reactions mainly consist of oxidation, reduction, and hydrolysis. During phase I metabolism, new polar functional groups, like hydroxyl or carboxyl groups, are introduced into the parent molecules, which results in either excretion of the modified chemical with the urine or in further metabolism by phase II metabolic reactions. During phase II metabolism (i.e., conjugation reactions), chemicals are conjugated with endogenous hydrophilic molecules (e.g., glucuronic acid, sulfate, glycine, and acetyl group), which strongly increases their hydrophilicity and facilitates their excretion. Metabolism can also influence the biological activity of a chemical. In most cases, metabolism works as a detoxification system, as it can convert biologically active chemicals into less active or even inactive metabolites [11]. In contrast, some chemicals that have no initial biological activity can be metabolically activated to a biologically active chemical (i.e., prodrugs) [12]. The principle of prodrugs is often used in the pharmaceutical industry, with the aim being to improve the pharmacokinetics of drugs [13]. For example, enalapril is a medication that is used for the treatment of arterial hypertension, and in the body, it is metabolized by esterases to the pharmacologically active compound enalaprilat [14]. Additionally, some chemicals can be metabolized to reactive metabolites, as seen for the thiophene moiety [12], and can have detrimental effects.

Thus, metabolism can strongly influence the endocrine activities of many chemicals. Rybacka and coworkers developed an in silico model for the prediction of endocrine-disrupting potential of industrial chemicals and their metabolites [15]. More than 6000 industrial chemicals were evaluated using this model, and 9% of them were predicted to be positive for interactions with the ER. However, when metabolism was incorporated into this model, this doubled the number of chemicals that were defined as positive for interactions with the ER [15]. Metabolism can, for example, significantly affect antiestrogenic and antiandrogenic activities of the new

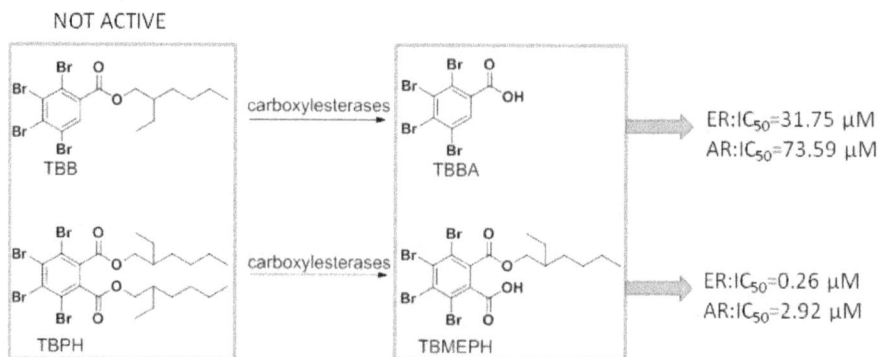

Figure 1.
Metabolism of the new brominated flame retardants TBB and TBPH to their TBBA and TBMEPH metabolites that show antiestrogenic and antiandrogenic activities, as determined using a yeast assay [16]. ER, estrogen receptor; AR, androgen receptor.

brominated flame retardants 2-ethylhexyl 2,3,4,5-tetrabromobenzoate (TBB) and bis(2-ethylhexyl) tetrabromophthalate (TBPH). While these parent chemicals show no activity toward ERs and androgen receptors, their metabolites 2,3,4,5-tetrabromobenzoic acid (TBBA) and 2-ethylhexyltetrabromobenzoate ester (TBMEPH) show antiestrogenic and antiandrogenic activities with IC_{50} values in the low micromolar (**Figure 1**) [16].

However, as *in vitro* assays do not generally consider metabolic transformations of chemicals, it can be difficult to detect chemicals without estrogenic activities that are converted to metabolites with estrogenic activities (i.e., proestrogens). Moreover, *in vitro* estrogenic activities can be overestimated for compounds that are metabolized to inactive metabolites *in vivo* [17]. This can result in poor *in vitro* to *in vivo* predictions, as observed with benzyl-butyl phthalate, which has estrogenic activity in the T47D-KBluc *in vitro* assay, but not in the *in vivo* uterotrophic assay. This can be explained by the rapid hydrolysis of benzyl-butyl phthalate to its monoester *in vivo*, which has no estrogenic activity [9]. In contrast, methoxychlor metabolites have higher estrogenic activity than methoxychlor itself, which is why the *in vivo* estrogenic activity for methoxychlor is higher than that predicted from *in vitro* assays (**Figure 2**) [9].

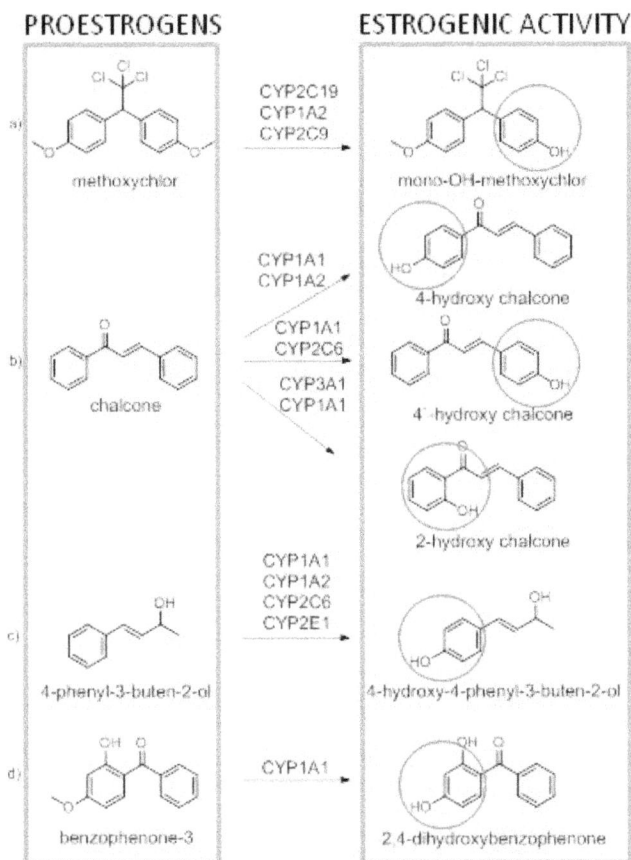

Figure 2.
Metabolism of proestrogens to active metabolites with estrogenic activity. In all of these examples, hydroxylation at the para position of the aromatic ring is responsible for the estrogenic activity.

2. Metabolism of 17β-estradiol

17β-Estradiol (E2) metabolism has been extensively studied, especially in connection with risk of premenopausal breast cancer [18, 19]. E2 can undergo aromatic hydroxylation that is catalyzed by cytochromes P450, for the C2 and C4 positions of the steroid rings, to form catechol structures, or for the C16 position of the steroid rings, to form 16-hydroxyestrone structures [20]. Estrogen metabolites with a catechol structure are further metabolized by catechol-O-methyltransferase to their methylated metabolites, as shown in **Figure 3**. The 16-hydroxyestrones are further metabolized to 17-epiestriols and estriols (**Figure 3**). As determined in the urine of premenopausal women, *in vivo* the 16-hydroxylation pathway of estradiol metabolism is the most important, followed by the 2-hydroxylation pathway, while the 4-hydroxylation pathway represents only minor metabolic conversion [20].

Different environmental factors and polymorphic variations in the genes that encode metabolic enzymes have also been reported to affect estradiol metabolism [24]. Smoking and high physical activity, for example, both favor the 2-hydroxylation metabolic pathway, with the 16-hydroxylation pathway decreased [25, 26]. Moreover, Gu and coworkers reported on connections between smoking and increased metabolism of estradiol, increased activity of the 4-hydroxylation metabolic pathway, and decreased methylation of estrogen metabolites [25].

The catechol estrogens 2-hydroxyestradiol and 4-hydroxyestradiol can bind to the ER of MCF-7 cells, and their relative binding activities compared to E2 were reported to be 23 and 26%, respectively [27]. These work as agonists of ER-dependent gene expression in the MCF-7 cell line [28].

The estrogenic activities of E2 and its metabolites were evaluated in luciferase reporter gene assays using T47D breast cancer cells (i.e., the ER-CALUX assay) [21]. The estrogenic activities of the E2 metabolites were compared with that of E2, which can be represented as the "E2 equivalency factor" (EEF) (**Figure 3**). E2 was the most potent compound, while its metabolites had reduced estrogenic

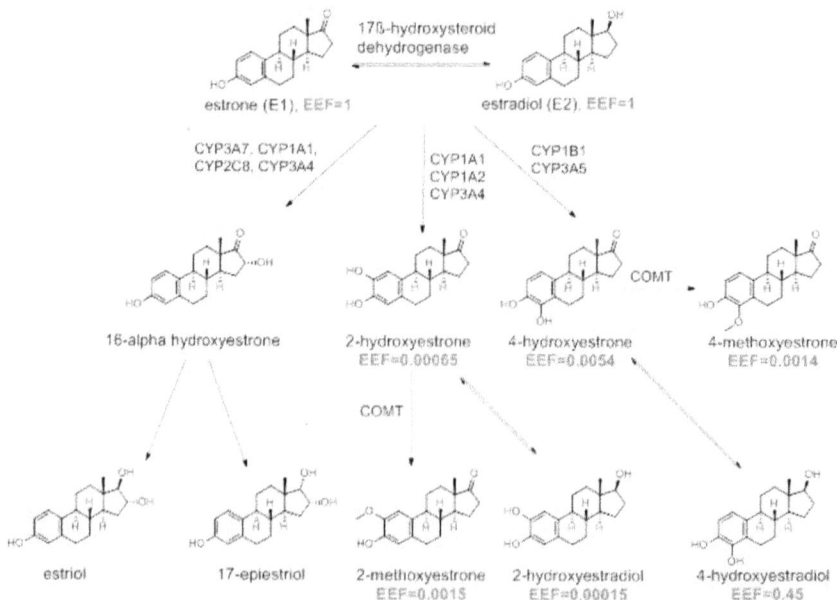

Figure 3.
Endogenous metabolism of E2 together with the E2 equivalency factors (EEF) for the various metabolites, as determined with the ER-CALUX assay [20–23]. COMT, catechol-O-methyltransferase.

activities. Here, the 4-hydroxy metabolites, and especially 4-hydroxyestradiol, had higher estrogenic activities than the 2-hydroxy metabolites [21]. Both of these forms of hydroxylated estradiols (i.e., 4-hydroxyestradiol, 2-hydroxyestradiol) increased uterine weight of neonatal rats, which confirmed their estrogenic activities *in vivo* [29]. 4-Hydroxyestradiol had greater *in vivo* estrogenic activity than 2-hydroxyestradiol (203, 107% increases in uterine weight, respectively) [29].

3. Impact of metabolism on estrogenic activity

As mentioned above, metabolites with altered estrogenic activity can be formed during metabolism. In some cases, estrogenic activities can be predicted from the structures of the metabolites. Some structural characteristics of the molecule are known to be important for binding to the ER, such as the aromatic ring with an OH group at the *para* position [30]. Hydroxylation of the *para* position of the aromatic ring, which is a common phase I metabolic reaction, often enhances estrogenicity. In contrast, glucuronides are devoid of estrogenic activity.

3.1 Metabolic activation of proestrogens

A number of chemicals that have been reported to be without estrogenic activities *in vitro* can affect the estrogen system *in vivo*. Methoxychlor is a broad-spectrum pesticide, and as such it is one of the most studied proestrogens. While methoxychlor has no estrogenic activity, its mono-demethylated and bis-demethylated metabolites have significant estrogenic activities [31]. Mollergues et al. determined the estrogenic activity of methoxychlor using the ER-CALUX assay with and without the β-naphthoflavone-/phenobarbital-induced S9 fraction [32]. In this assay, methoxychlor showed weak estrogenic activity (EC_{50} 4.6 μM). This estrogenic activity was significantly increased when the activated S9 fraction was added to the assay (EC_{50} 0.15 μM), which suggested the formation of active metabolites of methoxychlor. The pure methoxychlor metabolite 4,4'-(2,2,2-trichloroethane-1,1-diyl) diphenol was also tested, and its estrogenic activity was comparable with that of methoxychlor treated with the S9 fraction (EC_{50} 0.05 μM), which suggested that 4,4'-(2,2,2-trichloroethane-1,1-diyl) diphenol is the main metabolite formed with the S9 fraction [32]. As the methoxychlor metabolites mono-OH methoxychlor and bis-OH-methoxychlor are formed both *in vitro* and *in vivo*, addition of the metabolic enzymes here (i.e., the S9 fraction) improved the *in vivo* prediction [33]. Additionally, Sumida and coworkers added a source of metabolic enzymes (i.e., human and rat S9 and liver microsomes) to MCF-7 and Hela reporter gene assays to determine the influence of metabolism on the estrogenic activity of trans-stilbene and methoxychlor [33]. While these parent compounds were without estrogenic activities, the addition of the metabolic enzymes resulted in significant increases in estrogenicity [33].

Chalcone is an α,β-unsaturated ketone, and it is a structural fragment in many natural chemicals. Chalcone itself is without estrogenic activity. However, estrogenic activities were shown for its hydroxylated metabolites using a luciferase reporter assay with the MCF-7 cell line (**Figure 2**) [34]. Similarly, CYP-mediated hydroxylation on the aromatic ring of 4-phenyl-3-buten-2-ol results in estrogenic activity of its 4-hydroxyl metabolite (**Figure 2**) [34]. Benzophenone-3 is a widely used UV filter in sunscreens. While the estrogenic activity of benzophenone-3 determined with a reporter assay using CHO cells was weak, its main metabolite 2,4-dihydroxybenzophenone showed >20-fold ERα agonist activity (EC_{50} 2.2, 0.099 μM, respectively) and 100-fold ERβ agonist activity (EC_{50} 3.3, 0.033 μM, respectively) (**Figure 2**) [35]. This enhanced estrogenicity is, however, not surprising, as a 4-hydroxyl group on the phenol ring is essential for strong estrogenic activity.

Permethrin and bifenthrin are pyrethroid pesticides [36]. In *in vitro* reporter gene assays using the BG-1 cell line (i.e., CALUX bioassays), neither of them showed ER agonist activity, while bifenthrin acted as an ER antagonist. However, both of these pesticides induced expression of chloriogenin (i.e., an E2-responsive protein) in *in vivo* assays in the juvenile fish *Menidia beryllina*, which indicated estrogenic activities for both of the parent pesticides or their metabolites *in vivo* [36].

These differences between the *in vitro* and *in vivo* data for permethrin might be due to the formation of metabolites with higher estrogenic activities [37, 38]. Similarly, a higher estrogenic activity of the parent bifenthrin that was shown in an *in vivo* study was also seen for the bifenthrin metabolites [39].

3.2 Metabolic inactivation

Inconsistencies in the estrogenic activities obtained *in vitro* and *in vivo* were also seen for different phthalates [40]. Here, the tested phthalates (i.e., *n*-butyl benzyl phthalate, dicyclohexyl phthalate, 2-ethylhexyl phthalate, di-*n*-butyl phthalate) showed estrogenic activities in an *in vitro* MCF-7 proliferation assay (i.e., the E-screen assay), but they did not induce expression of calbindin-D_{9K} mRNA *in vivo* in neonatal rat uterus [40]. The explanation here might lie in the rapid *in vivo* metabolism of phthalates to monoester metabolites, which have no estrogenic activity [41]. *n*-Butyl benzyl phthalate is rapidly metabolized to mono-*n*-butyl phthalate, mono-benzyl phthalate, hippuric acid, phthalic acid, and benzoic acid [42]. In two *in vitro* assays (i.e., E-screen assay, progesterone receptor assay on MCF-7 cell line), *n*-butyl benzyl phthalate showed estrogenic activities, while its metabolites were without activity (**Figure 4**) [42].

Loss of estrogenic activity has also been described for various glucuronides. For example, the soy isoflavones genistein and daidzein are known as estrogens [43]. In contrast, their glucuronides are not estrogenic [44]. Despite this, glucuronides have shown very low estrogenic activities in *in vitro* reporter gene assays using U2OS cells (~0.002–0.0005-fold that of their aglycones), which can be explained by their intracellular deconjugation to their corresponding aglycones [44]. Beekmann and

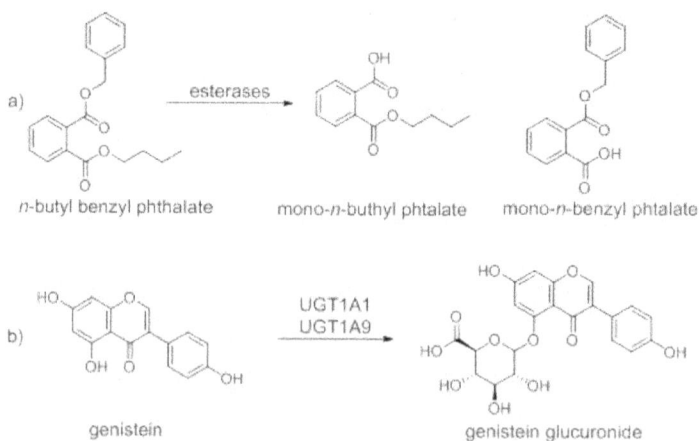

a)

n-butyl benzyl phthalate   esterases →   mono-*n*-buthyl phtalate   mono-*n*-benzyl phtalate

b)

genistein   UGT1A1 UGT1A9 →   genistein glucuronide

Figure 4.
Metabolism of the estrogenic compounds n-butyl benzyl phthalate to its inactive monoester metabolites (a) and genistein to the inactive genistein glucuronide (b).

coworkers used a cell-free microarray assay for real-time co-regulator-nuclear receptor interactions, which enabled the detection of estrogenicity as an agonistic response to the ER ligand-binding domain (LBD) [45]. They reported 0.125-fold to 0.00022-fold potencies for the glucuronides in comparison with their corresponding aglycones for the modulation of ERα-LBD and ERβ-LBD-co-regulator interactions [45].

Similarly, *in vitro* estrogenic activities were shown for *p*-nonylphenol and *p*-octylphenol with yeast cells, with EC_{50} values in the high nanomolar range (EC_{50} 110, 700 nM, respectively) [46]. Their glucuronides were without agonistic and antagonistic estrogenic and androgenic activities [46]. Due to the rapid glucuronidation of *p*-nonylphenol and *p*-octylphenol *in vivo*, these *in vitro* estrogenicities probably do not reflect any hazards *in vivo* [46].

4. Bisphenols

The bisphenols are chemicals that contain two phenol rings that are connected through a bridging atom, which can be a carbon or a sulfur, as for BPA and bisphenol S (BPS; bis(4-hydroxyphenyl)sulfone), respectively [47]. BPA is the best known bisphenol as it is used as a monomer in the production of polycarbonate plastic and epoxy resins, and it is also known to be an endocrine disruptor [16, 48–54]. Both the metabolism and endocrine effects of BPA have been studied in detail, although there remains a lack of information on some of its analogs.

For the bisphenols, their metabolism has a protecting role. Their conjugation with glucuronic acid and sulfate is the main *in vivo* transformation for all of the bisphenols. In contrast to BPA as an agonist for the ERs, BPA glucuronide is without estrogenic activity [55]. Similar situations have been defined for the other bisphenol glucuronides, such as BPS glucuronide [56] and BPAF glucuronide [11]. A lack of estrogenic activity has also been shown for BPA sulfate [57]. In contrast to these conjugates, which are the main metabolites of the bisphenols, numerous oxidative metabolites of BPA have been detected. However, these were mainly reported for *in vitro* studies, whereas *in vivo* only hydroxylated BPA has been detected in feces in mice [58] and rats [59]. The estrogenic activity of the main BPA oxidative metabolite is lower than that of BPA [60]. Among the oxidative metabolites, two have shown significantly greater estrogenic activities than BPA: its *ipso* metabolite 4-methyl-2,4-bis(p-hydroxyphenyl)pent-1-ene (MBP) and hydroxycumyl alcohol. The MBP estrogenic activity has been determined in several *in vitro* and *in vivo* assays, in which it has shown up to 500-fold estrogenic activity over BPA (**Figure 5**, **Table 1**) [16, 62–65]. Additionally, hydroxycumyl alcohol has shown ∼100-fold estrogenic activity over BPA [66]. However, there are questions about the *in vivo* relevance of these data. Indeed, although MBP has very high estrogenic activity, it has not been detected *in vivo*, as BPA glucuronidation is a much faster metabolic reaction *in vivo*.

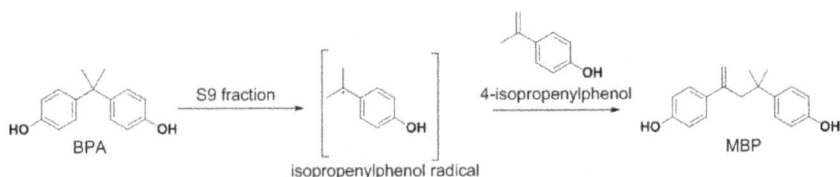

Figure 5.
BPA metabolic activation through formation of the potent estrogenic metabolite MBP [61].

Assay system	EC$_{50}$ (μM)		Relative potency	Reference
	MBP	BPA	(MBP *vs* BPA)	
Yeast reporter assay	0.014	3.6	257	[16]
MCF7-luc	0.0011	0.52	473	[63]
ERE-luc in NIH3T3 cells	0.00068	1.0	1470	[63]
Yeast two-hybrid assay	0.0083	14	1686	[63]
Yeast estrogen screen assay	0.71	160	225	[63]
Uterotrophic assay	NR	NR	500	[65]
Vitellogenin induction	NR	NR	250	[64]

Table 1.
Estrogenic agonistic activity of MBP compared to BPA, according to various in vitro and in vivo assays [61].

Hashimoto and coworkers evaluated the estrogenic activity of 13 BPA-related compounds using a yeast two-hybrid system without and with the addition of an S9 fraction [67]. Most of these chemicals showed enhanced estrogenic activities when the S9 fraction was added. This might be explained by the formation of oxidative metabolites with enhanced estrogenic activities [61]. A similar situation was reported for bisphenol B (BPB; 2,2-bis(4-hydroxyphenyl)butane), which is a more potent ER agonist than BPA [60]. Metabolism can also affect this BPB estrogenic activity. Here, after incubation of BPB with an S9 fraction, there was enhanced estrogenicity, which was probably due to the formation of BPB dimers [62, 68]. Nevertheless, *in vivo*, glucuronidation is the predominant metabolic pathway for the bisphenols, while their oxidative metabolites are in most cases detected only *in vitro*.

5. Testing strategies

In vitro systems for evaluation of estrogenic activity are usually limited to target chemicals, without taking into account that many chemicals are extensively metabolized, which can have significant effects on their estrogenic activities. For some of the cell lines used for endocrine testing, metabolic activities have been confirmed. However, for reliable data, it is important that the metabolic capacity of any *in vitro* system is in good agreement with the *in vivo* conditions, although that can be difficult to ascertain. Bursztyka and coworkers [69] evaluated the metabolic capacities toward the known endocrine disruptors genistein and BPA for various cell lines that are commonly used in endocrine testing (i.e., the HepG2, MCF7, and HC11 cell lines) [69]. Phase I metabolic activities were not seen for these tested cell lines. The HepG2 and MCF7 cell lines showed glucuronidation and sulfation activities toward genistein and BPA, while the HC11 cell line was without metabolic activity. However, phase II metabolism in these cell lines was not representative of *in vivo* conditions. So, while sulfate conjugates of genistein and BPA were the main metabolites detected in these cell lines, it is known that genistein and BPA are mainly metabolized to glucuronide conjugates *in vivo* [69].

Testing strategies that include metabolic aspects have not been well defined. While different approaches can be used, they generally have many drawbacks. Jacobsen et al. [70] used two approaches: a compound-by-compound approach and an effects-based approach (**Figure 6**) [70].

In the compound-by-compound approach, the relevant metabolites are identified, isolated or synthesized, and then evaluated for their endocrine activities, together with the parent chemical. Moreover, mixtures of a parent chemical and its metabolites can be tested, to determine the effects of such mixtures (e.g., synergism, additive, and antagonistic). This approach is commonly used [16, 56, 63, 71]. A drawback to this approach is that there is a need to conduct metabolic studies, as in many cases the metabolites are not known. Additionally, *in vitro* studies of metabolism can result in a "pallet" of metabolites, where not all will be relevant *in vivo* [61].

In the effects approach, the endocrine activity of the parent chemical is compared to the endocrine activity of the parent chemical treated with a metabolizing system, which is usually an S9 fraction [70]. Incorporation of such metabolic systems into *in vitro* assays is a common practice when testing for genotoxicity, like for the Ames test, where the S9 fraction is added as a source of metabolic enzymes, although such metabolic systems are still rarely used for the evaluation of endocrine activities of different chemicals [72].

In a recent study, a rat S9 fraction was incorporated in a CALUX reporter gene assay (i.e., the U2-OS cell line), and 27 chemicals were evaluated [73]. Selective inclusion of cofactors enables the evaluation of the different phases of metabolism on the estrogenic activities (i.e., phase I, nicotinamide adenine dinucleotide *phosphate [reduced]*; phases I and II, nicotinamide adenine dinucleotide *phosphate [reduced]*, UDP-glucuronic acid, phosphoadenosylphosphosulfate, glutathione). These data showed that the endocrine activities for 23 of the 27 chemicals tested

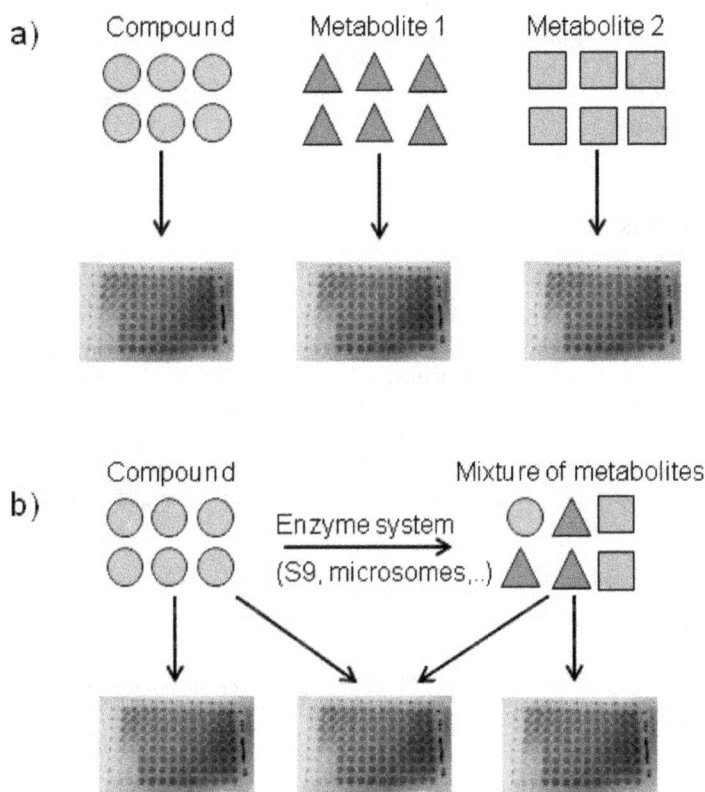

Figure 6.
Testing strategies that include metabolic aspects. The compound-by-compound approach (a) and the effects approach (b), as proposed by Jacobsen and coworkers [70].

were affected by metabolism. Phase II metabolism resulted in decreased estrogenic activities, which is expected and is in agreement with *in vivo* data. For example, BPA and genistein showed lower estrogenic activities after phase II metabolism. In contrast, after phase I metabolism, 5 of the chemicals showed lower estrogenic activities, and 11 of the chemicals showed higher estrogenic activities [73].

However, also the effects approach has many weaknesses, as, for example, the metabolites formed *in vitro* are not necessarily formed *in vivo*. These data should therefore be interpreted with caution. The optimal path might therefore be the inclusion of both strategies (i.e., chemical by chemical, effects approach) [70]. Moreover, Jacobsen and coworkers proposed a five-step scheme for the evaluation of the endocrine effects of chemicals and their metabolites [70]:

1. The endocrine activity of the parent chemical should be determined. Then, based on all of the available information, an *in vitro* metabolizing system for the production of the metabolites should be selected (e.g., S9 fractions, microsomes, as the most common systems).

2. The compatibility of the metabolizing system and the test system for determination of the endocrine activities should then be evaluated.

3. The mixture of metabolites formed with the metabolizing system should then be evaluated for endocrine activity.

4. The influence of the metabolite mixture on the endocrine activity of the parent chemical should then be evaluated.

5. The endocrine activities of the pure metabolites and their mixtures should then be evaluated.

6. Conclusions

Metabolism is considered as a detoxification system that lowers biological activities and facilitates excretion of foreign chemicals. This appears to be true for many estrogenic chemicals, including E2, which is metabolized to numerous metabolites that have significantly lower estrogenic activities. However, some chemicals that are without estrogenic activity can be metabolized to potent estrogens. Some metabolic pathways in particular, such as hydroxylation on the *para* position of the aromatic ring, are dangerous in terms of the metabolic activation of proestrogens. Metabolic aspects should therefore be considered when testing chemicals for estrogenic activities.

Acknowledgements

This study was supported by the Slovenian Research Agency (Grant Nos. Programme P1-0208 and Programme P1-0245).

Conflict of interest

The authors declare that they have no conflicts of interest.

Author details

Darja Gramec Skledar and Lucija Peterlin Mašič*
Faculty of Pharmacy, University of Ljubljana, Ljubljana, Slovenia

*Address all correspondence to: lucija.peterlin@ffa.uni-lj.si

IntechOpen

References

[1] Damstra T, Barlow S, Bergman A, Kavlock R, Van Der Kraak G. Global Assessment of the State-of-the-Science of Endocrine Disruptors. Geneva: World Health Organisation; 2002. pp. 1-180

[2] Rochester JR. Bisphenol A and human health: A review of the literature. Reproductive Toxicology. 2013;**42**:132-155

[3] Kabir ER, Rahman MS, Rahman I. A review on endocrine disruptors and their possible impacts on human health. Environmental Toxicology and Pharmacology. 2015;**40**(1):241-258

[4] Acconcia F, Pallottini V, Marino M. Molecular mechanisms of action of BPA. Dose-Response. 2015;**13**(4): 1559325815610582

[5] Usman A, Ahmad M. From BPA to its analogues: Is it a safe journey? Chemosphere. 2016;**158**:131-142

[6] Welshons WV, Nagel SC, vom Saal FS. Large effects from small exposures. III. Endocrine mechanisms mediating effects of bisphenol A at levels of human exposure. Endocrinology. 2006;**147**(6): 56-69

[7] Svobodová K, Cajthaml T. New *in vitro* reporter gene bioassays for screening of hormonal active compounds in the environment. Applied Microbiology and Biotechnology. 2010;**88**(4):839-847

[8] Gelbke HP, Kayser M, Poole A. OECD test strategies and methods for endocrine disruptors. Toxicology. 2004; **205**(1–2):17-25

[9] Conley JM, Hannas BR, Furr JR, Wilson VS, Gray LE. A demonstration of the uncertainty in predicting the estrogenic activity of individual chemicals and mixtures from an *in vitro* estrogen receptor transcriptional activation assay (T47D-KBluc) to the *in vivo* uterotrophic assay using oral exposure. Toxicological Sciences. 2016; **153**(2):382-395

[10] Gramec Skledar D, Troberg J, Lavdas J, Peterlin Mašič L, Finel M. Differences in the glucuronidation of bisphenols F and S between two homologous human UGT enzymes, 1A9 and 1A10. Xenobiotica. 2015;**45**(6): 511-519

[11] Li M, Yang YJ, Yang Y, Yin J, Zhang J, Feng YX, et al. Biotransformation of Bisphenol AF to its major glucuronide metabolite reduces estrogenic activity. PLoS One. 2013;**8**(12)

[12] Gramec D, Peterlin Mašič L, Sollner Dolenc M. Bioactivation potential of thiophene-containing drugs. Chemical Research in Toxicology. 2014;**27**(8): 1344-1358

[13] Zawilska JB, Wojcieszak J, Olejniczak AB. Prodrugs: A challenge for the drug development. Pharmacological Reports. 2013;**65**(1):1-14

[14] MacFadyen RJ, Meredith PA, Elliott HL. Enalapril clinical pharmacokinetics and pharmacokinetic-pharmacodynamic relationships. An overview. Clinical Pharmacokinetics. 1993;**25**(4):274-282

[15] Rybacka A, Rudén C, Tetko IV, Andersson PL. Identifying potential endocrine disruptors among industrial chemicals and their metabolites—Development and evaluation of in silico tools. Chemosphere. 2015;**139**:372-378

[16] Fic A, Zegura B, Gramec D, Mašič LP. Estrogenic and androgenic activities of TBBA and TBMEPH, metabolites of novel brominated flame retardants, and selected bisphenols, using the XenoScreen XL YES/YAS assay. Chemosphere. 2014;**112**:362-369

[17] Soto AM, Maffini MV, Schaeberle CM, Sonnenschein C. Strengths and weaknesses of *in vitro* assays for estrogenic and androgenic activity. Best Practice & Research. Clinical Endocrinology & Metabolism. 2006; **20**(1):15-33

[18] Brinton LA, Trabert B, Anderson GL, Falk RT, Felix AS, Fuhrman BJ, et al. Serum estrogens and estrogen metabolites and endometrial cancer risk among postmenopausal women. Cancer Epidemiology, Biomarkers & Prevention. 2016;**25**(7):1081-1089

[19] Ziegler RG, Fuhrman BJ, Moore SC, Matthews CE. Epidemiologic studies of estrogen metabolism and breast cancer. Steroids. 2015;**99**:67-75

[20] Eliassen AH, Ziegler RG, Rosner B, Veenstra TD, Roman JM, Xu X, et al. Reproducibility of fifteen urinary estrogens and estrogen metabolites over a 2- to 3-year period in premenopausal women. Cancer Epidemiology, Biomarkers & Prevention. 2009;**18**(11): 2860-2868

[21] Hoogenboom LAP, de Haan L, Hooijerink D, Bor G, Murk AJ, Brouwer A. Estrogenic activity of estradiol and its metabolites in the ER-CALUX assay with human T47D breast cells. APMIS. 2001;**109**(2):101-107

[22] Ziegler RG, Rossi SC, Fears TR, Bradlow HL, Adlercreutz H, Sepkovic D, et al. Quantifying estrogen metabolism: An evaluation of the reproducibility and validity of enzyme immunoassays for 2-hydroxyestrone and 16alpha-hydroxyestrone in urine. Environmental Health Perspectives. 1997;**105**(3):607-614

[23] Tsuchiya Y, Nakajima M, Yokoi T. Cytochrome P450-mediated metabolism of estrogens and its regulation in human. Cancer Letters. 2005;**227**(2):115-124

[24] Samavat H, Kurzer MS. Estrogen metabolism and breast cancer. Cancer Letters. 2015;**356**:231-243

[25] Gu F, Caporaso NE, Schairer C, Fortner RT, Xu X, Hankinson SE, et al. Urinary concentrations of estrogens and estrogen metabolites and smoking in caucasian women. Cancer Epidemiology, Biomarkers & Prevention. 2013;**22**(1):58-68

[26] Matthews CE, Fortner RT, Xu X, Hankinson SE, Eliassen AH, Ziegler RG. Association between physical activity and urinary estrogens and estrogen metabolites in premenopausal women. The Journal of Clinical Endocrinology and Metabolism. 2012;**97**(10):3724-3733

[27] Schütze N, Vollmer G, Wünsche W, Grote A, Feit B, Knuppen R. Binding of 2-hydroxyestradiol and 4-hydroxyestradiol to the estrogen receptor of MCF-7 cells in cytosolic extracts and in nuclei of intact cells. Experimental and Clinical Endocrinology. 1994;**102**(5):399-408

[28] Schütze N, Vollmer G, Knuppen R. Catecholestrogens are agonists of estrogen receptor dependent gene expression in MCF-7 cells. The Journal of Steroid Biochemistry and Molecular Biology. 1994;**48**(5–6):453-461

[29] Newbold RR, Liehr JG. Induction of uterine adenocarcinoma in CD-1 mice by catechol estrogens. Cancer Research. 2000;**60**(2):235-237

[30] Devillers J, Marchand-Geneste N, Carpy A, Porcher JM. SAR and QSAR modeling of endocrine disruptors. SAR and QSAR in Environmental Research. 2006;**17**(4):393-412

[31] Kupfer D, Bulger WH. Metabolic activation of pesticides with proestrogenic activity. Federation Proceedings. 1987;**46**(5):1864-1869

[32] Mollergues J, van Vugt-Lussenburg B, Kirchnawy C, Bandi RA, van der Lee RB, Marin-Kuan M, et al. Incorporation of a metabolizing system in biodetection assays for endocrine active substances. ALTEX. 2016;**34**(3):389-398

[33] Sumida K, Ooe N, Nagahori H, Saito K, Isobe N, Kaneko H, et al. An *in vitro* reporter gene assay method incorporating metabolic activation with human and rat S9 or liver microsomes. Biochemical and Biophysical Research Communications. 2001;**280**(1):85-91

[34] Kohno Y, Kitamura S, Sanoh S, Sugihara K, Fujimoto N, Ohta S. Metabolism of the alpha,beta-unsaturated ketones, chalcone and trans-4-phenyl-3-buten-2-one, by rat liver microsomes and estrogenic activity of the metabolites. Drug Metabolism and Disposition. 2005;**33**(8):1115-1123

[35] Watanabe Y, Kojima H, Takeuchi S, Uramaru N, Sanoh S, Sugihara K, et al. Metabolism of UV-filter benzophenone-3 by rat and human liver microsomes and its effect on endocrine-disrupting activity. Toxicology and Applied Pharmacology. 2015;**282**(2):119-128

[36] Brander SM, He G, Smalling KL, Denison MS, Cherr GN. The *in vivo* estrogenic and *in vitro* anti-estrogenic activity of permethrin and bifenthrin. Environmental Toxicology and Chemistry. 2012;**31**(12):2848-2855

[37] McCarthy AR, Thomson BM, Shaw IC, Abell AD. Estrogenicity of pyrethroid insecticide metabolites. Journal of Environmental Monitoring. 2006;**8**(1):197-202

[38] Nillos MG, Chajkowski S, Rimoldi JM, Gan J, Lavado R, Schlenk D. Stereoselective biotransformation of permethrin to estrogenic metabolites in fish. Chemical Research in Toxicology. 2010;**23**(10):1568-1575

[39] DeGroot BC, Brander SM. The role of P450 metabolism in the estrogenic activity of bifenthrin in fish. Aquatic Toxicology. 2014;**156**:17-20

[40] Hong EJ, Ji YK, Choi KC, Manabe N, Jeung EB. Conflict of estrogenic activity by various phthalates between *in vitro* and *in vivo* models related to the expression of Calbindin-D9k. The Journal of Reproduction and Development. 2005;**51**(2):253-263

[41] Okubo T, Suzuki T, Yokoyama Y, Kano K, Kano I. Estimation of estrogenic and anti-estrogenic activities of some phthalate diesters and monoesters by MCF-7 cell proliferation assay *in vitro*. Biological & Pharmaceutical Bulletin. 2003;**26**(8):1219-1224

[42] Picard K, Lhuguenot JC, Lavier-Canivenc MC, Chagnon MC. Estrogenic activity and metabolism of n-butyl benzyl phthalate *in vitro*: Identification of the active molecule(s). Toxicology and Applied Pharmacology. 2001; **172**(2):108-118

[43] Vitale DC, Piazza C, Melilli B, Drago F, Salomone S. Isoflavones: Estrogenic activity, biological effect and bioavailability. European Journal of Drug Metabolism and Pharmacokinetics. 2013;**38**(1):15-25

[44] Islam MA, Bekele R, Van den Berg JH, Kuswanti Y, Thapa O, Soltani S, et al. Deconjugation of soy isoflavone glucuronides needed for estrogenic activity. Toxicology *In Vitro*. 2015; **29**(4):706-715

[45] Beekmann K, de Haan LH, Actis-Goretta L, Houtman R, van Bladeren PJ, Rietjens IM. The effect of glucuronidation on isoflavone induced estrogen receptor (ER)α and ERβ mediated coregulator interactions. The Journal of Steroid Biochemistry and Molecular Biology. 2015;**154**:245-253

[46] Moffat GJ, Burns A, Van Miller J, Joiner R, Ashby J. Glucuronidation of nonylphenol and octylphenol eliminates their ability to activate transcription via the estrogen receptor. Regulatory Toxicology and Pharmacology. 2001; **34**(2):182-187

[47] Schmidt J, Masic LP. Organic synthetic environmental endocrine disruptors: Structural classes and metabolic fate. Acta Chimica Slovenica. 2012;**59**(4):722-738

[48] Krishnan AV, Stathis P, Permuth SF, Tokes L, Feldman D. Bisphenol-A: An estrogenic substance is released from polycarbonate flasks during autoclaving. Endocrinology. 1993;**132**(6):2279-2286

[49] Perez P, Pulgar R, Olea-Serrano F, Villalobos M, Rivas A, Metzler M, et al. The estrogenicity of bisphenol A-related diphenylalkanes with various substituents at the central carbon and the hydroxy groups. Environmental Health Perspectives. 1998;**106**(3):167-174

[50] Yamasaki K, Sawaki M, Takatsuki M. Immature rat uterotrophic assay of bisphenol A. Environmental Health Perspectives. 2000;**108**(12):1147-1150

[51] Markey CM, Michaelson CL, Veson EC, Sonnenschein C, Soto AM. The mouse uterotrophic assay: A reevaluation of its validity in assessing the estrogenicity of bisphenol A. Environmental Health Perspectives. 2001;**109**(1):55-60

[52] Chen MY, Ike M, Fujita M. Acute toxicity, mutagenicity, and estrogenicity of bisphenol-A and other bisphenols. Environmental Toxicology. 2002;**17**(1): 80-86

[53] Richter CA, Birnbaum LS, Farabollini F, Newbold RR, Rubin BS, Talsness CE, et al. *In vivo* effects of bisphenol A in laboratory rodent studies. Reproductive Toxicology. 2007; **24**(2):199-224

[54] Wetherill YB, Akingbemi BT, Kanno J, McLachlan JA, Nadal A, Sonnenschein C, et al. *In vitro* molecular mechanisms of bisphenol A action. Reproductive Toxicology. 2007;**24**(2): 178-198

[55] Snyder RW, Maness SC, Gaido KW, Welsch F, Sumner SC, Fennell TR. Metabolism and disposition of bisphenol A in female rats. Toxicology and Applied Pharmacology. 2000;**168**(3): 225-234

[56] Skledar DG, Schmidt J, Fic A, Klopcic I, Trontelj J, Dolenc MS, et al. Influence of metabolism on endocrine activities of bisphenol S. Chemosphere. 2016;**157**:152-159

[57] Shimizu M, Ohta K, Matsumoto Y, Fukuoka M, Ohno Y, Ozawa S. Sulfation of bisphenol A abolished its estrogenicity based on proliferation and gene expression in human breast cancer MCF-7 cells. Toxicology *In Vitro*. 2002; **16**(5):549-556

[58] Zalko D, Soto AM, Dolo L, Dorio C, Rathahao E, Debrauwer L, et al. Biotransformations of bisphenol A in a mammalian model: Answers and new questions raised by low-dose metabolic fate studies in pregnant CD1 mice. Environmental Health Perspectives. 2003;**111**(3):309-319

[59] Knaak JB, Sullivan LJ. Metabolism of bisphenol A in the rat. Toxicology and Applied Pharmacology. 1966;**8**(2): 175-184

[60] Kitamura S, Suzuki T, Sanoh S, Kohta R, Jinno N, Sugihara K, et al. Comparative study of the endocrine-disrupting activity of bisphenol A and 19 related compounds. Toxicological Sciences. 2005;**84**(2):249-259

[61] Gramec Skledar D, Peterlin Mašič L. Bisphenol A and its analogs: Do their metabolites have endocrine activity? Environmental Toxicology and Pharmacology. 2016;47:182-199

[62] Yoshihara S, Makishima M, Suzuki N, Ohta S. Metabolic activation of bisphenol A by rat liver S9 fraction. Toxicological Sciences. 2001;62(2): 221-227

[63] Yoshihara S, Mizutare T, Makishima M, Suzuki N, Fujimoto N, Igarashi K, et al. Potent estrogenic metabolites of bisphenol A and bisphenol B formed by rat liver S9 fraction: Their structures and estrogenic potency. Toxicological Sciences. 2004;78(1):50-59

[64] Ishibashi H, Watanabe N, Matsumura N, Hirano M, Nagao Y, Shiratsuchi H, et al. Toxicity to early life stages and an estrogenic effect of a bisphenol A metabolite, 4-methyl-2,4-bis(4-hydroxyphenyl)pent-1-ene on the medaka (*Oryzias latipes*). Life Sciences. 2005;77(21):2643-2655

[65] Okuda K, Takiguchi M, Yoshihara S. *In vivo* estrogenic potential of 4-methyl-2,4-bis(4-hydroxyphenyl)pent-1-ene, an active metabolite of bisphenol A, in uterus of ovariectomized rat. Toxicology Letters. 2010;197(1):7-11

[66] Nakamura S, Tezuka Y, Ushiyama A, Kawashima C, Kitagawara Y, Takahashi K, et al. *Ipso* substitution of bisphenol A catalyzed by microsomal cytochrome P450 and enhancement of estrogenic activity. Toxicology Letters. 2011;203(1):92-95

[67] Hashimoto Y, Moriguchi Y, Oshima H, Kawaguchi M, Miyazaki K, Nakamura M. Measurement of estrogenic activity of chemicals for the development of new dental polymers. Toxicology *In Vitro*. 2001;15(4–5): 421-425

[68] Okuda K, Fukuuchi T, Takiguchi M, Yoshihara S. Novel pathway of metabolic activation of bisphenol A-related compounds for estrogenic activity. Drug Metabolism and Disposition. 2011;39(9):1696-1703

[69] Bursztyka J, Perdu E, Pettersson K, Pongratz I, Fernandez-Cabrera M, Olea N, et al. Biotransformation of genistein and bisphenol A in cell lines used for screening endocrine disruptors. Toxicology *In Vitro*. 2008;22(6): 1595-1604

[70] Jacobsen NW, Brooks BW, Halling-Sørensen B. Suggesting a testing strategy for possible endocrine effects of drug metabolites. Regulatory Toxicology and Pharmacology. 2012;62(3):441-448

[71] Kang JS, Choi JS, Kim WK, Lee YJ, Park JW. Estrogenic potency of bisphenol S, polyethersulfone and their metabolites generated by the rat liver S9 fractions on a MVLN cell using a luciferase reporter gene assay. Reproductive Biology and Endocrinology. 2014;12:102

[72] Jacobs MN, Janssens W, Bernauer U, Brandon E, Coecke S, Combes R, et al. The use of metabolising systems for *in vitro* testing of endocrine disruptors. Current Drug Metabolism. 2008;9(8): 796-826

[73] van Vugt-Lussenburg BMA, van der Lee RB, Man HY, Middelhof I, Brouwer A, Besselink H, et al. Incorporation of metabolic enzymes to improve predictivity of reporter gene assay results for estrogenic and anti-androgenic activity. Reproductive Toxicology. 2018;75:40-48

Chapter 3

Estrogen for Male Function: Effect of Changes in the Sex Hormone Milieu on Erectile Function

Tomoya Kataoka and Kazunori Kimura

Abstract

Androgens are essential for male physical activity and normal erectile function. Moreover, estrogens also influence erectile function, and high estrogen levels are a risk factor for erectile dysfunction (ED). In this review, we summarize relevant research examining the effects of the sex hormone milieu on erectile function. Testosterone affects several organs, particularly erectile tissue. The mechanisms through which testosterone deficiency affects erectile function and the results of testosterone replacement therapy have been extensively studied. Estrogen, the female sexual hormone, also affects erectile function, as demonstrated in both clinical and basic studies. Interestingly, estradiol-testosterone imbalance is considered a risk factor for ED. Furthermore, endocrine-disrupting chemicals have estrogen-like effects and cause ED. Phosphodiesterase-5 (PDE-5) inhibitors, first-line drugs for the treatment of ED, increase the levels of testosterone and estradiol in patients with low testosterone levels. Therefore, estrogen levels should be carefully monitored in patients receiving PDE-5 inhibitors. Future studies are needed to confirm these findings using molecular tools in order to provide insights into the treatment and mechanisms of endocrine-related ED.

Keywords: estrogen, testosterone, endocrine-disrupting chemical, phosphodiesterase-5 inhibitor, erectile dysfunction, endothelial function

1. Introduction

Serum estrogen levels are correlated with symptoms of aging in men, and estrogen may therefore play an important role in aging [1, 2]. Several previous studies have suggested that estrogen levels may also affect erectile function [3–6]. Indeed, older and obese men have been found to have not only low androgen levels but also high estrogen levels. Since testosterone is metabolized to estradiol by aromatase, the particularly high aromatase levels in visceral adipose tissue may explain the elevated estradiol levels among obese men [7]. Visceral adipose tissue often accumulates among men with increasing age. Interestingly, high estrogen levels have been observed in older patients who present with a lack of sexual interest and erectile dysfunction (ED); therefore, these symptoms in the elderly are thought to involve a pathophysiological estrogen-testosterone imbalance [6, 8–10].

Accordingly, in this review, we discuss the effects of sex hormone imbalances on male erectile function.

2. Erectile function and sexual hormones

There are many reports on erectile function and sexual hormones. Erectile function is controlled by complex mechanisms [11], including the vascular and nervous systems [12–16]. One of the most important materials is a nitric oxide (NO). After NO is releasing in the penis, corporal smooth muscle relaxes. However, when NO production is decreased, the erectile function weakened, resulting in ED. The relaxant system is also important for the erectile function. The relaxant system is controlled by both the endothelial and the nervous systems. When the upper stream of smooth muscle relaxant system is weakened, ED is caused; therefore, many studies have focused on smooth muscle relaxation. In contrast, corporal smooth muscle contraction is controlled by constrictors, such as noradrenaline in the flaccid state. However, if the contraction be upregulated in some situations, ED would be caused.

Interestingly, some studies have indicated that smooth muscle relaxation and contraction balance is disturbed by abnormal activation of contractile signaling pathway such as the adrenergic regulation. In some syndromes causing ED, such as diabetes mellitus or metabolic syndrome, the contraction is enhanced [17–19]. One of the important contractile signaling pathways is the RhoA/Rho-kinase signaling pathway. The enhancement is known to occur in aged individuals. The inhibition of RhoA/Rho-kinase signaling pathway by Y-27632 has been shown to improve ED in aged animal models [20, 21]. Interestingly, the contractility of smooth muscle in the corpus cavernosum is regulated by sexual hormones and may play a significant role in erectile function.

3. Testosterone deficiency and ED

Testosterone deficiency and ED have been studied extensively [22–25]. Testosterone deficiency causes ED using castrated animal models [26]. Furthermore, the erectile function is discussed by the endothelial NO synthase (eNOS) and neuronal NOS (nNOS) signalings. In some studies, testosterone administration to the castrated animals improved NOS expression in the penis and restored the erectile function [27]. Li et al. showed that testosterone deficiency decreases the upregulating reactive oxygen species production and it decreased eNOS activity (the phospho-eNOS/eNOS ratio) [28]. They also showed the reduction in eNOS activity induced cGMP levels decreased in the penis. Testosterone also alters phosphodiesterase type 5 (PDE-5) expression in the penis. Traish et al. showed that testosterone deficiency decreases PDE-5 activity using the rabbit model [29]. Additionally, Zhang et al. showed that PDE-5 expression was decreased by castration in the rat corpus cavernosum and that testosterone replacement therapy to the rats improved the expression [30]. These results indicate that testosterone is important for regulating PDE-5 expression. Traish et al. also suggested testosterone regulates not only NOS but also PDE-5 [31].

Testosterone also affects the smooth muscle of the corpus cavernosum. Reilly et al. reported that testosterone deficiency reduces the number of α-adrenergic-1 receptors in the castrated rats' smooth fascia [32]. Moreover, testosterone modulates the adrenergic response of the corpus cavernosum vascular smooth muscle [33]. These results indicate that when testosterone levels decrease, smooth muscle contractility also decreases. On the other hand, Sopko et al. showed that the levels of RhoA and Rho-kinase proteins are increased in the castrated rats' corpus cavernosum [34]. Their results indicated that testosterone deficiency increased smooth muscle contractility, leading to the decreasing erectile function and hypertension. Thus, although testosterone deficiency may increase contraction, additional research is required to more fully elucidate its impact on smooth muscle contraction.

Interestingly, testosterone also directly affects smooth muscle relaxation. Using isometric tension analysis, Yue et al. showed that the smooth muscle of rabbit coronary arteries and aortas are relaxed by testosterone [35]. Others have also reported that testosterone activates smooth muscle ATP-sensitive K^+ channels and regulates the relax response of the smooth muscles [36]. These findings indicate that testosterone may regulate erectile function locally by acting on corpus cavernosum smooth muscle. These results indicate that testosterone may affect both genomic and nongenomic mechanisms of erectile function.

Testosterone also affects the structure of the penis. For example, castrated rats exhibit smooth muscle loss and fibrosis [37], and testosterone deficiency increases the volume of collagen in the internal pudendal arteries [38]. These effects of testosterone indicate that testosterone deficiency causes programmed trabecular smooth muscle cell death (apoptosis) [29]. Traish et al. also indicated that testosterone deficiency is related to the accumulation of fat-containing cells (fibroblasts or preadipocyte-like cells), particularly in the penis [39]. Interestingly, Wang et al. showed that testosterone deficiency decreases erectile function and increases collagen in the corporeal cavernosum by inhibiting autophagy and promoting apoptosis of the smooth muscle cells in rats' penis [40]. Although their report had several limitations, they discussed the important role of testosterone in regulating the structural integrity of the corpus cavernosum and erectile function. This resulted from testosterone regulating the counterregulation of autophagy and apoptosis by modulating the interactions between BECN1 and Bcl-2 (key dual regulators of autophagy and apoptosis) [41, 42].

4. Estrogen and ED in clinical studies

Estrogen, the female sex hormone, also affects erectile function. Interestingly, Tivesten et al. reported that that circulating free testosterone is positively associated with the ankle-brachial index (ABI) in a large population-based cohort of elderly males. They show that testosterone has a negative association with the degree of atherosclerotic disease in the lower extremities [43]. On the other hand, estrogen also has association with ABI negatively in the males, leading to higher estradiol levels associated with increased atherosclerosis. Besides, when lower extremity peripheral arterial disease (PAD) was defined as an ABI of less than 0.90, they showed that low serum testosterone and high serum estradiol are associated with lower extremity PAD. Moreover, both low testosterone levels and elevated estradiol levels affect erectile function and are associated with increased ED severity when present individually or concomitantly [44]. Low testosterone levels were thought to be the main effector; however, the presence of concomitantly elevated estradiol levels increased the severity of ED in patients with low testosterone levels. These reports indicated that female sex hormones also affect male health. Srilatha and Adaikan demonstrated that estradiol-testosterone imbalance is a risk factor for ED [8, 45, 46]. They showed that higher levels of estradiol were present in older patients experiencing with lack of sexual interest and ED, after adjustment for age [8]. Additionally, they concluded that the estradiol-testosterone hormonal balance may be a determinant of successful management outcomes for ED. Wu et al. also reported an association between sexual dysfunction and changes in estradiol and testosterone levels in Chinese men [47], and O'Connor et al. reported that estradiol was associated with sexual function-related distress; higher levels were related to greater distress in 2838 men, ages 40–79 years, who completed the European Male Aging Study-Sexual Function Questionnaire [48]. These reports specifically demonstrated the relationship between high estrogen milieu and male erectile function.

Serum estrogen levels are controlled by aromatase but can be altered under some conditions. Lamba et al. reported that antiretroviral therapy is associated with sexual dysfunction and increased serum estradiol levels in men [49]. Moreover, they found that total estradiol levels may be increased based on sex hormone-binding globulin (SHBG) levels. Drugs such as phenytoin are known to cause elevations in serum estradiol and SHBG [50]. Increased levels of SHBG, for example, due to induction of aromatase or SHBG synthetase, lead to a decrease in the free androgen index. Additionally, increased levels of SHBG and/or a low free androgen index have been associated with hypertension, osteoporosis, varicose veins, sexual dysfunction, and adverse serum lipids [51–56]. All these side effects have been reported in association with antiretroviral therapy as well. SHBG, similar to other globulins, is upregulated in patients with acquired immunodeficiency syndrome and human immunodeficiency virus infection [57, 58]. Hassan et al. have also reported the association of overhydration with male sexual dysfunction and depression in hemodialysis patients [59]. They showed that overhydration in hemodialysis patients was associated with a higher prevalence of sexual dysfunction and depression, lower serum levels of total testosterone and dehydroepiandrosterone, and higher levels of serum estradiol. Intriguingly, Tivesten et al. reported that circulating estradiol is a predictor of the progression of carotid artery intima-media thickness in middle-aged men [60]. They also reported that elderly men with low serum testosterone and estradiol have increased risk of mortality and that patients with low testosterone and estradiol levels have the highest risk of mortality [61]. Serum estrogen levels can be altered by some drugs and sex hormones. Therefore, ED induced by high estrogen may be related to mortality.

5. Estrogen and ED in basic research

Interestingly, estrogen administration decreases erectile function in animal models [62, 63]. Researchers administered estradiol orally to rats, resulting in high estradiol levels and low testosterone levels. Moreover, the intracavernous pressure (ICP) response to nerve stimulation was also impaired in all treated groups, and trichrome staining demonstrated the presence of cavernosal connective tissue hyperplasia in long-term study groups [62]. Oral administration of estradiol to rabbits resulted in high estradiol levels and low testosterone levels, similar to the effects in rats. Additionally, acetylcholine induced endothelium-mediated relaxation in normal animals, but this effect was significantly attenuated in treated groups, and NO-mediated nonadrenergic, noncholinergic neurotransmission was decreased in the treatment groups [63].

In our previous studies, subcutaneous administration (s.c.) of estradiol to rats resulted in high estradiol levels and low testosterone levels, thereby decreasing erectile function [64]. Moreover, we administered testosterone to rats with high estrogen-induced testosterone deficiency; however, erectile function did not improve. Interestingly, estrogen administration increases the contraction of smooth muscle in the corpus cavernosum, upregulating the RhoA/Rho-kinase signaling pathway, which is involved in ED [18]. Vignozzi et al. demonstrated that high-fat diet-induced ED is associated with high estradiol levels, rather than low testosterone levels [65].

We also investigated the influence of estradiol-testosterone imbalance on erectile function in rats (**Figures 1–6; Table 1**). Male Wistar ST rats (11 weeks old, Japan SLC Inc., Hamamatsu, Japan) were separated into five groups. In the low testosterone (Low-T) group (n = 11), rats were injected with goserelin (LH-RH agonist, 0.9 mg/kg, s.c.). In the low testosterone and high estrogen (Low-T/High-E) group (n = 11), rats were injected with goserelin and estradiol (3 μg/kg/day, s.c.) daily from weeks 2 to 4. In the high estrogen (High-E) group (n = 11), rats were injected with estradiol daily from weeks 2 to 4. In the high estrogen and testosterone (High-E/High-T) group (n = 11), rats were injected with estradiol and testosterone (3 mg/kg/day, s.c.) daily from weeks 2 to 4. In the control group (n = 11), rats were not injected with any hormone. **Table 1** shows the sex hormone concentrations in rats. Goserelin injection significantly decreased serum bioavailable testosterone (control: 1.20 ± 0.13 ng/mL, Low-T: 0.55 ± 0.04 ng/mL, $P < 0.01$ versus the control; Low-T/High-E: 0.73 ± 0.06 ng/mL, $P < 0.05$ versus the control). Testosterone injection significantly increased serum bioavailable testosterone (control: 1.20 ± 0.13 ng/mL, High-E/High-T: 2.58 ± 0.31 ng/mL, $P < 0.001$ versus the control). Estradiol injection significantly increased serum estrogen (control: 102.5 ± 8.7 pg./mL, Low-T/High-E: 275.4 ± 34.4 pg./mL, $P < 0.01$ versus the control; High-E: 332.3 ± 17.4 pg./mL, $P < 0.001$ versus the control; High-E/High-T: 401.5 ± 51.6 pg./mL, $P < 0.001$ versus the control).

Figure 2 shows the erectile response to electrical field stimulation of the cavernous nerve in the different experimental groups. Analysis of the ICP/MAP ratio revealed that the ratios in the Low-T (0.52 ± 0.03), Low-T/High-E (0.46 ± 0.03), High-E (0.44 ± 0.03), and High-E/High-T (0.44 ± 0.02) groups, which represented

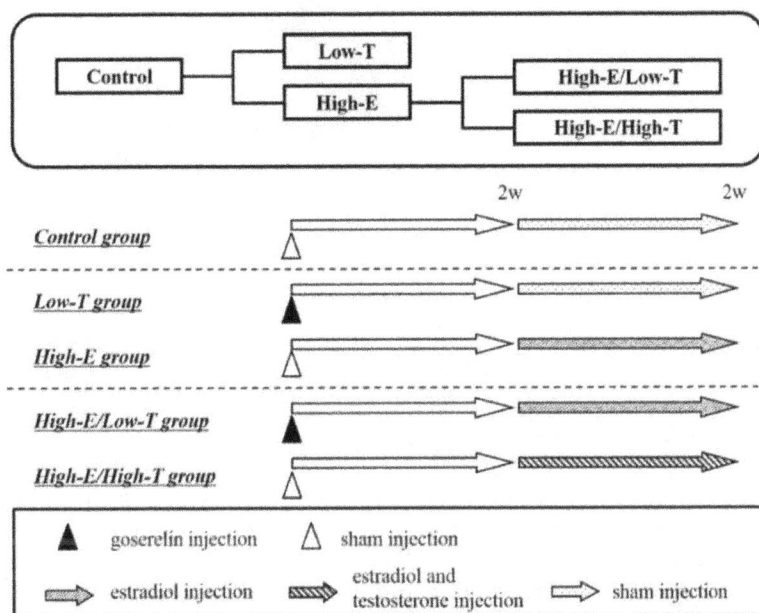

Figure 1.
Experimental design. In the control group, rats were injected with vehicle for 2 weeks. In the Low-T and High-E groups, rats were injected with goserelin acetate (LH-RH agonist, 0.9 mg/kg subcutaneously) at day 0. In the estrogen-treated (High-E) group, rats were injected with estradiol (3 mg/kg/day subcutaneously) for 2 weeks. In the estrogen- and testosterone-treated (High-E/High-T) group, rats were injected with estradiol (3 mg/kg/day subcutaneously) and testosterone (3 mg/kg/day subcutaneously) for 2 weeks. At the end of the period, rats were underwent erectile function testing in vivo or in vitro.

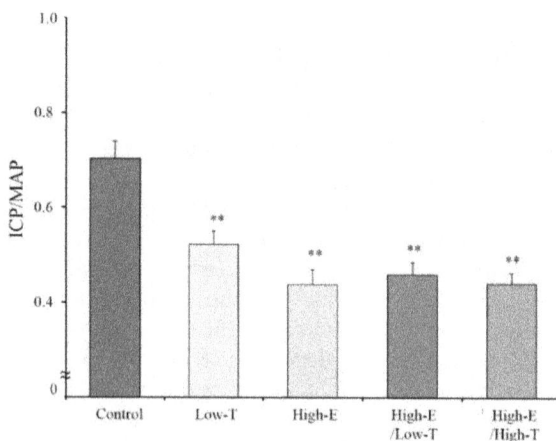

Figure 2.
Measurement of intracavernous pressure (ICP). Maximum ICP changes during electrical stimulation of the cavernous nerve in the control, Low-T, High-E, High-E/Low-T, and High-E/High-T groups. Data represent the means ± standard errors of the means (n = 6 per group). **P < 0.01 versus the control group by analysis of variance and Bonferroni-type multiple t-tests.

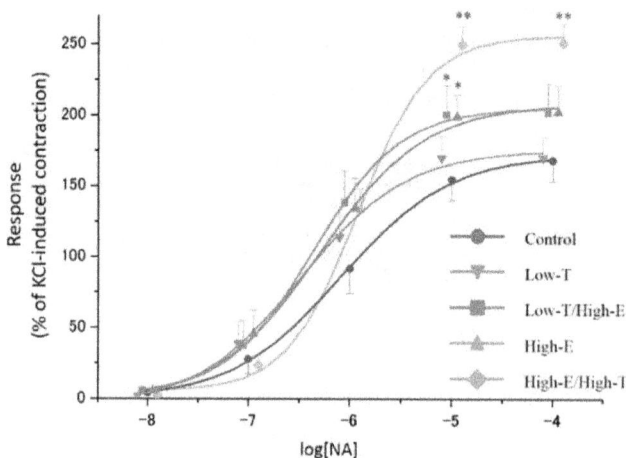

Figure 3.
The contraction curves induced by noradrenaline (NA) in rat corpus cavernosum strips. The contractile tone induced by 80 mM KCl was taken as 100%. Data reported in all graphs represent the means ± standard errors of the means (n = 5 per group). *P < 0.05, **P < 0.01 versus the control group by analysis of variance and Bonferroni-type multiple t-tests. Emax values are reported in the text.

all treated rats, were significantly lower than in the control group (0.70 ± 0.04, $P < 0.01$). These data suggested that erectile responses were decreased in rats with a sex hormone imbalance.

Figure 3 shows the contractile response of rat corpora cavernosa strips to increasing concentrations of noradrenaline (NA). Increasing concentrations of NA were found to contract rat corpora cavernosa strips in all groups. In particular, 10 µM NA resulted in statistically significant differences in the in vitro penile contractile response among the experimental groups (control: 154.5 ± 14.1%, Low-T: 169.8 ± 14.8%, Low-T/High-E: 200.2 ± 21.1%, High-E: 198.9 ± 15.3%, High-E/High-T: 249.7 ± 13.5%). Although the contractile response did not differ between the control

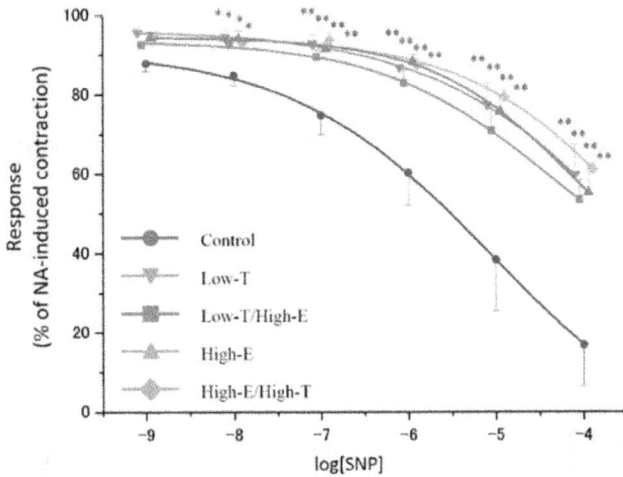

Figure 4.
*The relaxation curve induced by sodium nitroprusside (SNP) in rat corpus cavernosum strips. The strips were precontracted using 10^{-5} M NA. Data reported in all graphs represent the means ± standard errors of the means (n = 5 per group). *P < 0.05, **P < 0.01 versus the control group by analysis of variance and Bonferroni-type multiple t-tests. Emax values are reported in the text.*

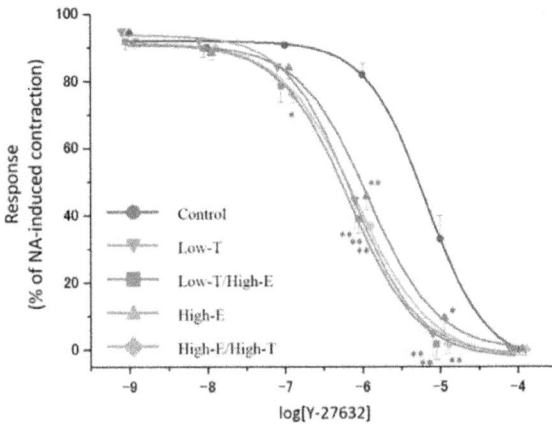

Figure 5.
*The relaxation curves induced by Rho-kinase inhibitor Y-27632 in rat corpus cavernosum strips. The strips were precontracted using 10^{-5} M NA. Data reported in all graphs represent the means ± standard errors of the means (n = 5 per group). *P < 0.05, **P < 0.01 versus the control group by analysis of variance and Bonferroni-type multiple t-tests. IC_{50} values are reported in the text.*

group and the Low-T group ($P > 0.05$), the contractile responses in the Low-T/High-E, High-E, and High-E/High-T groups were higher than the response in the control group ($P < 0.05$).

Figures 4 and **5** show the relaxant response of NA-precontracted rat corpora cavernosa strips to increasing concentrations of sodium nitroprusside (SNP) and Y-27632. In all groups, increasing concentrations of the NO donor SNP relaxed rat corpora cavernosa strips (control: Emax = 16.8 ± 10.3%, Low-T: Emax = 59.7 ± 7.6%, Low-T/High-E: Emax = 53.4 ± 5.0%, High-E: Emax = 55.2 ± 6.8%, High-E/High-T: Emax = 61.1 ± 1.5%). In the treated groups, the sensitivities to SNP were significantly lower than in the control group ($P < 0.01$). Increasing concentrations of

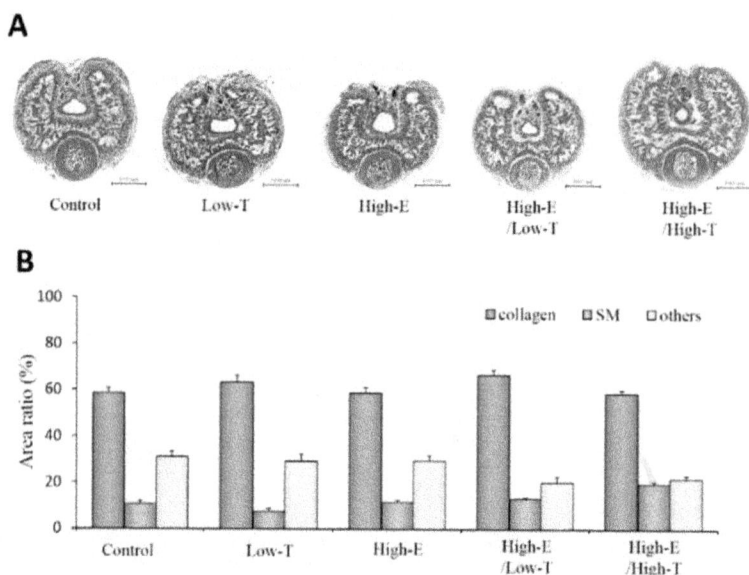

A

| Control | Low-T | High-E | High-E /Low-T | High-E /High-T |

B

Figure 6.
The rat penis sections of Masson's trichrome staining. (A) Representative specimens of corpus cavernosum of each group rats. (B) Histological evaluation of the tissues. The area ratios of the collagen fibers, smooth muscle (SM), and others were calculated using computerized image analysis. Data reported in all graphs represent the means ± standard errors of the means (n = 3 per group).

	Bio-T (ng/mL)	Estrogen (pg/mL)
Control	1.20 ± 0.13	102.5 ± 8.7
Low-T	0.55 ± 0.04**	51.2 ± 4.2
High-E	0.90 ± 0.12	332.3 ± 17.4**
High-E/Low-T	0.73 ± 0.06*	275.4 ± 34.4**
High-E/High-T	2.58 ± 0.31**	401.5 ± 51.6**

Data are expressed as means ± standard errors of the means. *P < 0.05, **P < 0.01 versus the control group by analysis of variance and Bonferroni-type multiple t-tests (n = 6 per group).

Table 1.
Serum levels of estrogen and bioavailable testosterone (bio-T) in rats.

Rho kinase inhibitor Y-27632 completely relaxed rat corpora cavernosa strips in all groups (control: half-maximal inhibitory concentration [IC_{50}] = 1.22 × 10^{-6} M, Low-T: IC_{50} = 2.43 × 10^{-7} M, Low-T/High-E: IC_{50} = 1.31 × 10^{-7} M, High-E: IC_{50} = 2.26 × 10^{-7} M, High-E/High-T: IC_{50} = 1.25 × 10^{-7} M). When using 10^{-6} M and 10^{-5} M Y-27632, the sensitivities to Y-27632 in the treated groups were significantly lower than in the control group (P < 0.01); thus, the graphs for the treated groups were shifted to the left.

Figure 6 shows the histological analysis of the rats' corpora cavernosa. The area ratio of the cavernous smooth muscle was analyzed (control: 10.5 ± 1.4%, Low-T: 7.4 ± 1.1%, Low-T/High-E: 13.2 ± 0.4%, High-E: 11.6 ± 0.1%, High-E/High-T: 19.4 ± 1.1%). Similarly, the area ratio of the collagen fiber was analyzed (control: 58.4 ± 2.5%, Low-T: 63.2 ± 3.0%, Low-T/High-E: 66.5 ± 2.3%, High-E: 58.8 ± 2.2%, High-E/High-T: 58.7 ± 1.4%). No statistically significant differences between the experimental groups were observed in the overall area ratios of smooth muscle, collagen fiber, and other parameters according to χ^2 tests for independence (P > 0.05).

Overall, we demonstrated that changes in the sex hormone milieu affected erectile function in rats, and our hypothesis that the sex hormone imbalance associated with ED was supported by both in vivo and in vitro experiments using pharmacological tools.

6. Estrogen receptors (ERs) in erectile function

Several reports have suggested an association between ERs and ED. Schultheiss et al. have shown the ER distribution in the corpus cavernosum penis of adult humans [66]. Additionally, Dietrich et al. have demonstrated that the corpus cavernosum and corpus spongiosum smooth muscles were immunoreactive for the androgen receptor (AR), ER-α, and ER-β and that endothelial cells were negative for AR, sporadically positive for ER-α, and positive for ER-β [67]. Jesmin et al. have demonstrated that ER-α was predominantly localized in the sensory corpuscle of the glans penis [68]. On the bother hands, they also reported that the ER-β was localized around the neurovascular bundle, artery, and nerve [68]. Spyridopoulos et al. have shown that the potential antiapoptotic effects of estrogen were impaired by reduced ER-β expression, and loss of antiapoptotic genes in the rat corpus cavernosum was associated with the pathogenesis of ED [69]. These reports indicate that the ER exists in the corpus cavernosum and has various functions. Moreover, the ER has been reported to be altered under some conditions. Shirai et al. have demonstrated that vascular endothelial growth factor treatment restores erectile function through stimulation of the insulin-like growth factor system and *ER-β* gene at the mRNA and protein levels in the corpus cavernosum of diabetic rats [70–72]. They had shown the expression of *ER-β* mRNA in male rat aortas before and after balloon denudation injury. Interestingly, the expression of *ER-α* mRNA in vascular endothelial and smooth muscle cells was very low levels after injury; however, the expression of *ER-β* mRNA in vascular endothelial cells was high after injury. Thus, the vascular protective effects of estrogen on endothelial and smooth muscle cells were exclusively mediated by ER-β, not ER-α [73]. Shirai et al. also demonstrated that the functionally predominant form of ER in the rat corpus cavernosum was ER-β and that age-related alterations in ER-β expression were likely related to the pathogenesis of ED in older rats. Thus, they concluded that downregulation of sex hormone receptors in the corpus cavernosum of aging rats is associated with ED [74]. Goyal et al. demonstrated the influence of estrogen on the structure of the corpus cavernosum [75–79] and showed that exposure to antiandrogens induces permanent structural abnormalities, including accumulation of fat cells, loss of smooth muscle cells and sinusoids, and reduced thickness of connective tissue trabeculae and tunica albuginea in the corpora cavernosa [76]. They also demonstrated that the ER and AR mediate cavernous smooth muscle cell differentiation, as shown by downregulation of MYH11 expression at the mRNA and protein levels and by reduced immunohistochemical staining of smooth muscle alpha actin using rats [79]. Therefore, a high estrogen milieu and alterations in ER expression may affect erectile function.

7. Endocrine-disrupting chemicals and ED

Some endocrine-disrupting chemicals have physiological effects similar to those of estrogen. Bisphenol A (BPA) is a widely used endocrine-disrupting chemical that is thought to have adverse health effects [80]. BPA has been widely produced and used as a common ingredient in the manufacture of plastics. Humans are mainly exposed to BPA through ingestion of foods containing BPA, and increasing evidence supports its association with impaired male reproductive function [81]. Manfo et al. reported that BPA also decreases erectile function [82], and Li et al. showed that BPA-exposed workers had significantly increased risk of ED (odds ratio = 4.5, 95% confidence interval: 2.1–9.8) [83, 84]. Moon et al. were the first to report the influence of BPA on erectile function using animal model [85]. They observed thickening of tunica albuginea, subtunical deposition of fat, and decreased sinusoidal space with subsequent increases in trabecular smooth muscle content by histological analysis in BPA-treated animals and demonstrated endothelial dysfunction in BPA-treated rabbits. Kovanecz et al. also reported that BPA decreases nNOS and vascular endothelial growth factor expression in rats [86, 87]. In these reports, BPA-induced ED was similar to high estrogen-induced ED. Thus, the relationship between endocrine-disrupting chemicals and ED should be carefully considered.

8. ED treatment and estrogen

PDE-5 inhibitors are the first choice for patients with ED. Recently, some interesting papers on PDE-5 inhibitors and estrogen have been published. Greco et al. reported a reduction in estrogen levels in patients with ED after chronic exposure to tadalafil, a PDE-5 inhibitor, and a concomitant increase in the testosterone-estrogen ratio [88]. They also showed that increased testosterone-estrogen ratios were not related to increases in testosterone serum levels, but rather to the possible effects of tadalafil on aromatase activity. Aversa et al. also demonstrated that daily tadalafil decreases serum estradiol levels [9]. In contrast, Spitzer et al. have reported that the PDE-5 inhibitor sildenafil increased estradiol levels in 40 men (ages 40–70 years) with ED, despite increasing testosterone levels [89]. Additionally, several reports have demonstrated that PDE-5 inhibitors increase testosterone levels [90–96]. When testosterone is low, estradiol levels may also be low because testosterone is metabolized to estradiol by aromatase. PDE-5 inhibitors can increase not only testosterone but also estradiol in patients with low testosterone levels. Therefore, estrogen levels should be carefully monitored in patients receiving PDE-5 inhibitors.

9. Conclusions

The sex hormone milieu affects erectile function, and sex hormone imbalances, particularly low testosterone levels combined with high estrogen levels, cause ED. Interestingly, estradiol has protective effects on female health, but harmful effects on male erectile function. Overall, these results provide insights into the possible treatments of endocrine-related ED. Future research should confirm these findings in more specific experiments using molecular tools.

Conflict of interest

The authors declare no conflicts of interest.

Author details

Tomoya Kataoka[1] and Kazunori Kimura[1,2]*

1 Department of Clinical Pharmaceutics, Graduate School of Medical Sciences, Nagoya City University, Japan

2 Department of Hospital Pharmacy, Graduate School of Pharmaceutical Sciences, Nagoya City University, Japan

*Address all correspondence to: kkimura@med.nagoya-cu.ac.jp

IntechOpen

References

[1] Wang C, Nieschlag E, Swerdloff R, Behre HM, Hellstrom WJ, Gooren LJ, et al. Investigation, treatment and monitoring of late-onset hypogonadism in males. European Journal of Endocrinology. 2008;**159**:507-514

[2] Morales A, Buvat J, Gooren LJ, Guay AT, Kaufman JM, Tan HM, et al. Endocrine aspects of sexual dysfunction in men. Journal of Sexual Medicine. 2004;**1**:69-81

[3] Diaz-Arjonilla M, Schwarcz M, Swerdloff RS, Wang C. Obesity, low testosterone levels and erectile dysfunction. International Journal of Impotence Research. 2009;**21**:89-98

[4] Yassin A, Saad F, Gooren LJ. Metabolic syndrome, testosterone deficiency and erectile dysfunction never come alone. Andrologia. 2008;**40**:259-264

[5] Corona G, Mannucci E, Fisher AD, Lotti F, Petrone L, Balercia G, et al. Low levels of androgens in men with erectile dysfunction and obesity. Journal of Sexual Medicine. 2008;**5**:2454-2463

[6] Shabsigh R, Arver S, Channer KS, Eardley I, Fabbri A, Gooren L, et al. The triad of erectile dysfunction, hypogonadism and the metabolic syndrome. International Journal of Clinical Practice. 2008;**62**:791-798

[7] Cohen PG. The role of estradiol in the maintenance of secondary hypogonadism in males in erectile dysfunction. Medical Hypotheses. 1998;**50**:331-333

[8] Srilatha B, Adaikan PG, Chong YS. Relevance of oestradiol-testosterone balance in erectile dysfunction patients' prognosis. Singapore Medical Journal. 2007;**48**:114-118

[9] Greco EA, Pili M, Bruzziches R, Corona G, Spera G, Aversa A. Testosterone:Estradiol ratio changes associated with long-term tadalafil administration: A pilot study. Journal of Sexual Medicine. 2006;**3**:716-722

[10] Basar MM, Aydin G, Mert HC, Keles I, Caglayan O, Orkun S, et al. Relationship between serum sex steroids and aging male symptoms score and international index of erectile function. Urology. 2005;**66**:597-601

[11] Andersson KE, Wagner G. Physiology of penile erection. Physiological Reviews. 1995;**75**:191-236

[12] Hotta Y, Hattori M, Kataoka T, Ohno R, Mikumo M, Maeda Y, et al. Chronic vardenafil treatment improves erectile function via structural maintenance of penile corpora cavernosa in rats with acute arteriogenic erectile dysfunction. Journal of Sexual Medicine. 2011;**8**(3):705-711

[13] Hotta Y, Ohno R, Kataoka T, Mikumo M, Takahata Y, Ohno M, et al. Effects of chronic vardenafil treatment persist after end of treatment in rats with acute arteriogenic erectile dysfunction. Journal of Sexual Medicine. 2012;**9**(7):1782-1788

[14] Abe Y, Hotta Y, Okumura K, Kataoka T, Maeda Y, Kimura K. Temporal changes in erectile function and endothelium-dependent relaxing response of corpus cavernosal smooth muscle after ischemia by ligation of bilateral internal iliac arteries in the rabbit. Journal of Pharmacological Sciences. 2012;**120**(3):250-253

[15] Shiota A, Hotta Y, Kataoka T, Morita M, Maeda Y, Kimura K. Oral L-citrulline supplementation improves erectile function in rats with acute arteriogenic erectile dysfunction. Journal of Sexual Medicine. 2013;**10**(10):2423-2429

[16] Musicki B, Bhunia AK, Karakus S, Burnett AL. S-nitrosylation of NOS pathway mediators in the penis contributes to cavernous nerve injury-induced erectile dysfunction. International Journal of Impotence Research. 2018;**30**:108-116

[17] Wingard C, Fulton D, Husain S. Altered penile vascular reactivity and erection in the Zucker obese-diabetic rat. Journal of Sexual Medicine. 2007;**4**:348-363

[18] Morelli A, Chavalmane AK, Filippi S, Fibbi B, Silvestrini E, Sarchielli E, et al. Atorvastatin ameliorates sildenafil-induced penile erections in experimental diabetes by inhibiting diabetes-induced RhoA/Rho-kinase signaling hyperactivation. Journal of Sexual Medicine. 2009;**6**:91-106

[19] Wingard CJ, Moukdar F, Prasad RY, Cathey BL, Wilkinson L. Reversal of voltage-dependent erectile responses in the Zucker obese-diabetic rat by rosuvastatin-altered RhoA/Rho-kinase signaling. Journal of Sexual Medicine. 2009;**6**:269-278

[20] Rajasekaran H, White S, Baquir A, Wilkes N. Rho-kinase inhibition improves erectile function in aging male Brown-Norway rats. Journal of Andrology. 2005;**26**:182-188

[21] Jin L, Liu T, Lagoda GA, Champion HC, Bivalacqua TJ, Burnett AL. Elevated RhoA/Rho-kinase activity in the aged rat penis: Mechanism for age-associated erectile dysfunction. FASEB Journal. 2006;**20**:536-538

[22] Kataoka T, Kimura K. Testosterone and erectile function, a review of evidence from basic research. In: Sex Hormones in Neurodegenerative Processes and Diseases. London: IntechOpen; 2017. pp. 257-272

[23] Kataoka T, Hotta Y, Maeda Y, Kimura K. Assessment of androgen replacement therapy for erectile function in rats with type 2 diabetes mellitus by examining nitric oxide-related and inflammatory factors. Journal of Sexual Medicine. 2014;**11**(4):920-929

[24] Kataoka T, Hotta Y, Maeda Y, Kimura K. Testosterone deficiency causes endothelial dysfunction via elevation of asymmetric dimethylarginine and oxidative stress in castrated rats. Journal of Sexual Medicine. 2017;**14**(12):1540-1548

[25] Hotta Y, Shiota A, Kataoka T, Motonari M, Maeda Y, Morita M, et al. Oral L-citrulline supplementation improves erectile function and penile structure in castrated rats. International Journal of Urology. 2014;**21**(6):608-612

[26] Mills TM, Lewis RW, Stopper VS. Androgenic maintenance of inflow and veno-occlusion during erection in the rat. Biology of Reproduction. 1998;**59**:1413-1418

[27] Armagan A, Kim NN, Goldstein I, Traish AM. Dose-response relationship between testosterone and erectile function: Evidence for the existence of a critical threshold. Journal of Andrology. 2006;**27**:517-526

[28] Li R, Meng X, Zhang Y, Wang T, Yang J, Niu Y, et al. Testosterone improves erectile function through inhibition of reactive oxygen species generation in castrated rats. PeerJ. 2016;**4**:e2000

[29] Traish AM, Park K, Dhir V, Kim NN, Moreland RB, Goldstein I. Effects of castration and androgen replacement on erectile function in a rabbit model. Endocrinology. 1999;**140**:1861-1868

[30] Zhang XH, Morelli A, Luconi M, Vignozzi L, Filippi S, Marini M, et al. Testosterone regulates PDE5 expression and in vivo responsiveness to tadalafil

in rat corpus cavernosum. European Urology. 2005;**47**:409-416

[31] Traish AM, Goldstein I, Kim NN. Testosterone and erectile function: From basic research to a new clinical paradigm for managing men with androgen insufficiency and erectile dysfunction. European Urology. 2007;**52**:54-70

[32] Reilly CM, Stopper VS, Mills TM. Androgens modulate the alphaadrenergic responsiveness of vascular smooth muscle in the corpus cavernosum. Journal of Andrology. 1997;**18**:26-31

[33] Reilly CM, Lewis RW, Stopper VS, Mills TM. Androgenic maintenance of the rat erectile response via a non-nitric-oxide-dependent pathway. Journal of Andrology. 1997;**18**:588-594

[34] Sopko NA, Hannan JL, Bivalacqua TJ. Understanding and targeting the Rho kinase pathway in erectile dysfunction. Nature Reviews in Urology. 2014;**11**:622-628

[35] Yue P, Chatterjee K, Beale C, Poole-Wilson PA, Collins P. Testosterone relaxes rabbit coronary arteries and aorta. Circulation. 1995;**91**:1154-1160

[36] Han DH, Chae MR, Jung JH, So I, Park JK, Lee SW. Effect of testosterone on potassium channel opening in human corporal smooth muscle cells. Journal of Sexual Medicine. 2008;**5**:822-832

[37] Dai YT, Stopper V, Lewis R, Mills T. Effects of castration and testosterone replacement on veno-occlusion during penile erection in the rat. Asian Journal of Andrology. 1999;**1**:53-59

[38] Alves-Lopes RU, Neves KB, Silva MA, Olivon VC, Ruginsk SG, Antunes-Rodrigues J, et al. Functional and structural changes in internal pudendal arteries underlie erectile dysfunction induced by androgen deprivation. Asian Journal of Andrology. 2017;**19**:526-532

[39] Traish AM, Toselli P, Jeong SJ, Kim NN. Adipocyte accumulation in penile corpus cavernosum of the orchiectomized rabbit: A potential mechanism for veno-occlusive dysfunction in androgen deficiency. Journal of Andrology. 2005;**26**:242-248

[40] Wang XJ, Xu TY, Xia LL, Zhong S, Zhang XH, Zhu ZW, et al. Castration impairs erectile organ structure and function by inhibiting autophagy and promoting apoptosis of corpus cavernosum smooth muscle cells in rats. International Urology and Nephrology. 2015;**47**:1105-1115

[41] Lian J, Karnak D, Xu L. The Bcl-2-Beclin 1 interaction in (−)-gossypol-induced autophagy versus apoptosis in prostate cancer cells. Autophagy. 2010;**6**:1201-1203

[42] Kang R, Zeh HJ, Lotze MT, Tang D. The Beclin 1 network regulates autophagy and apoptosis. Cell Death and Differentiation. 2011;**18**:571-580

[43] Tivesten A, Mellström D, Jutberger H, Fagerberg B, Lernfelt B, Orwoll E, et al. Low serum testosterone and high serum estradiol associate with lower extremity peripheral arterial disease in elderly men. The MrOS Study in Sweden. Journal of the American College of Cardiology. 2007;**50**(11):1070-1076

[44] El-Sakka AI. Impact of the association between elevated oestradiol and low testosterone levels on erectile dysfunction severity. Asian Journal of Andrology. 2013;**15**(4):492-496

[45] Srilatha B, Adaikan PG. Oestrogen-androgen crosstalk in the pathophysiology of erectile dysfunction. Asian Journal of Andrology. 2003;**5**(4):307-313

[46] Srilatha B, Adaikan PG. Endocrine milieu and erectile dysfunction: Is oestradiol-testosterone imbalance, a risk factor in the elderly? Asian Journal of Andrology. 2011;**13**(4):569-573

[47] Wu F, Chen T, Mao S, Jiang H, Ding Q, Xu G. Levels of estradiol and testosterone are altered in Chinese men with sexual dysfunction. Andrology. 2016;**4**(5):932-938

[48] O'Connor DB, Lee DM, Corona G, Forti G, Tajar A, O'Neill TW, et al. The relationships between sex hormones and sexual function in middle-aged and older European men. Journal of Clinical Endocrinology and Metabolism. 2011;**96**(10):E1577-E1587

[49] Lamba H, Goldmeier D, Mackie NE, Scullard G. Antiretroviral therapy is associated with sexual dysfunction and with increased serum oestradiol levels in men. International Journal of STD and AIDS. 2004;**15**(4):234-237

[50] Heroz AG, Levesque LA, Drislane FW, Ronthal M, Schomer DL. Phenytoin-induced elevation of serum oestradiol and reproductive dysfunction in men with epilepsy. Epilepsin. 1991;**32**:550-553

[51] Gyllenborg J, Rasmussen SL, Borch-Johnsen K, Heitmann BL, Skakkebaek NE, Juul A. Cardiovascular risk factors in men: The role of gonadal steroids and sex hormone-binding globulin. Metabolism. 2001;**50**:882-888

[52] Legrand E, Hedde C, Gallois Y, et al. Osteoporosis in men: A potential role for the sex hormone binding globulin. Bone. 2001;**29**:90-95

[53] Scopacasa F, Horowitz M, Wishart JM, Morris HA, Chatterton BE, Need AG. The relation between bone density, free androgen index, and oestradiol in men 60 to 70 years old. Bone. 2000;**27**:145-149

[54] Ciardullo AV, Panico S, Bellati C, et al. High endogenous oestradiol is associated with increased venous distensibility and clinical evidence of varicose veins in menopausal women. Journal of Vascular Surgery. 2000;**32**:544-549

[55] Aversa A, Isidori AM, De Martino MU, et al. Androgens and penile erection: Evidence for a direct relationship between free testosterone and cavernous vasodilation in men with erectile dysfunction. Clinical Endocrinology. 2000;**53**:517-522

[56] Phillips GB, Jing TY, Laragh JH, Sealey JE. Serum sex hormone levels and renin-sodium profile in men with hypertension. American Journal of Hypertension. 1995;**8**:626-629

[57] Martin ME, Benassayag C, Amiel C, Canton P, Nunez EA. Alterations in the concentrations and binding properties of sex steroid binding protein and corticosteroid-binding globulin in HIV+ patients. Endocrinological Investigation. 1992;**15**:597-603

[58] Laudat A, Blum L, Guéchot J, Picard O, Cabane J, Imbert JC, et al. Changes in systemic gonadal and adrenal steroids in asymptomatic human inmmunodeficiency virus-infected men: Relationship with the CD4 cell counts. European Journal of Endocrinology. 1995;**133**:418-424

[59] Hassan K, Elimeleh Y, Shehadeh M, Fadi H, Rubinchik I. The relationship between hydration status, male sexual dysfunction and depression in hemodialysis patients. Therapeutics and Clinical Risk Management. 2018;**14**:523-529

[60] Tivesten A, Hulthe J, Wallenfeldt K, Wikstrand J, Ohlsson C, Fagerberg B. Circulating estradiol is an independent predictor of progression of carotid artery intima-media thickness

in middle-aged men. Journal of Clinical Endocrinology and Metabolism. 2006;**91**(11):4433-4437

[61] Tivesten A, Vandenput L, Labrie F, Karlsson MK, Ljunggren O, Mellström D, et al. Low serum testosterone and estradiol predict mortality in elderly men. Journal of Clinical Endocrinology and Metabolism. 2009;**94**(7):2482-2488

[62] Adaikan PG, Srilatha B. Oestrogen-mediated hormonal imbalance precipitates erectile dysfunction. International Journal of Impotence Research. 2003;**15**(1):38-43

[63] Srilatha B, Adaikan PG. Estrogen and phytoestrogen predispose to erectile dysfunction: Do ER-alpha and ER-beta in the cavernosum play a role? Urology. 2004;**63**(2):382-386

[64] Kataoka T, Hotta Y, Ohno M, Maeda Y, Kimura K. Limited effect of testosterone treatment for erectile dysfunction caused by high-estrogen levels in rats. International Journal of Impotence Research. 2013;**25**(6):201-205

[65] Vignozzi L, Filippi S, Comeglio P, Cellai I, Morelli A, Marchetta M, et al. Estrogen mediates metabolic syndrome-induced erectile dysfunction: A study in the rabbit. Journal of Sexual Medicine. 2014;**11**(12):2890-2902

[66] Schultheiss D, Badalyan R, Pilatz A, Gabouev AI, Schlote N, Wefer J, et al. Androgen and estrogen receptors in the human corpus cavernosum penis: Immunohistochemical and cell culture results. World Journal of Urology. 2003;**21**(5):320-324

[67] Dietrich W, Haitel A, Huber JC, Reiter WJ. Expression of estrogen receptors in human corpus cavernosum and male urethra. Journal of Histochemistry and Cytochemistry. 2004;**52**(3):355-360

[68] Jesmin S, Mowa CN, Matsuda N, Salah-Eldin AE, Togashi H, Sakuma I, et al. Evidence for a potential role of estrogen in the penis: Detection of estrogen receptor-alpha and -beta messenger ribonucleic acid and protein. Endocrinology. 2002;**143**(12):4764-4774

[69] Spyridopoulos I, Sullivan AB, Kearney M, Isner JM, Losordo DW. Estrogen-receptor-mediated inhibition of human endothelial cell apoptosis. Estradiol as a survival factor. Circulation. 1997;**95**(6):1505-1514

[70] Shirai M, Yamanaka M, Shiina H, Igawa M, Ogishima T, Fujime M, et al. Androgen, estrogen, and progesterone receptor gene regulation during diabetic erectile dysfunction and insulin treatment. Urology. 2004;**64**(6):1244-1249

[71] Shirai M, Yamanaka M, Shiina H, Igawa M, Kawakami T, Ishii N, et al. Vascular endothelial growth factor restores erectile function through modulation of the insulin-like growth factor system and sex hormone receptors in diabetic rat. Biochemical and Biophysical Research Communications. 2006;**341**(3):755-762

[72] Yamanaka M, Shirai M, Shiina H, Shirai M, Tanaka Y, Fujime M, et al. Loss of anti-apoptotic genes in aging rat crura. Journal of Urology. 2002;**168**(5):2296-2300

[73] Lindner V, Kim SK, Karas RH, Kuiper GG, Gustafsson JA, Mendelsohn ME. Increased expression of estrogen receptor-beta mRNA in male blood vessels after vascular injury. Circulation Research. 1998;**83**(2):224-229

[74] Shirai M, Yamanaka M, Shiina H, Igawa M, Fujime M, Lue TF, et al. Downregulation of androgen, estrogen and progesterone receptor genes and protein is involved in aging-related erectile dysfunction. International Journal of Impotence Research. 2003;**15**(6):391-396

[75] Goyal HO, Braden TD, Williams CS, Dalvi P, Williams JW, Srivastava KK. Exposure of neonatal male rats to estrogen induces abnormal morphology of the penis and loss of fertility. Reproductive Toxicology. 2004;18(2):265-274

[76] Simon L, Avery L, Braden TD, Williams CS, Okumu LA, Williams JW, et al. Exposure of neonatal rats to anti-androgens induces penile mal-developments and infertility comparable to those induced by oestrogens. International Journal of Andrology. 2012;35(3):364-376

[77] Goyal HO, Braden TD, Williams CS, Dalvi P, Mansour MM, Mansour M, et al. Abnormal morphology of the penis in male rats exposed neonatally to diethylstilbestrol is associated with altered profile of estrogen receptor-alpha protein, but not of androgen receptor protein: A developmental and immunocytochemical study. Biology of Reproduction. 2004;70(5):1504-1517

[78] Goyal HO, Braden TD, Cooke PS, Szewczykowski MA, Williams CS, Dalvi P, et al. Estrogen receptor alpha mediates estrogen-inducible abnormalities in the developing penis. Reproduction. 2007;133(5):1057-1067

[79] Okumu LA, Bruinton S, Braden TD, Simon L, Goyal HO. Estrogen-induced maldevelopment of the penis involves down-regulation of myosin heavy chain 11 (MYH11) expression, a biomarker for smooth muscle cell differentiation. Biology of Reproduction. 2012;87(5):109

[80] Dodds EC, Lawson W. Synthetic strogenic agents without the phenanthrene nucleus. Nature. 1936;137:996

[81] Yamada H, Furuta I, Kato EH, Kataoka S, Usuki Y, Kobashi G, et al. Maternal serum and amniotic fluid bisphenol A concentrations in the early second trimester. Reproductive Toxicology. 2002;16:735-739

[82] Manfo FP, Jubendradass R, Nantia EA, Moundipa PF, Mathur PP. Adverse effects of bisphenol A on male reproductive function. Reviews of Environmental Contamination and Toxicology. 2014;228:57-82

[83] Li D, Zhou Z, Qing D, He Y, Wu T, Miao M, et al. Occupational exposure to bisphenol-A (BPA) and the risk of self-reported male sexual dysfunction. Human Reproduction. 2010;25(2):519-527

[84] Li DK, Zhou Z, Miao M, He Y, Qing D, Wu T, et al. Relationship between urine bisphenol-A level and declining male sexual function. Journal of Andrology. 2010;31(5):500-506

[85] Moon DG, Sung DJ, Kim YS, Cheon J, Kim JJ. Bisphenol A inhibits penile erection via alteration of histology in the rabbit. International Journal of Impotence Research. 2001;13(5):309-316

[86] Kovanecz I, Gelfand R, Masouminia M, Gharib S, Segura D, Vernet D, et al. Chronic high dose intraperitoneal bisphenol A (BPA) induces substantial histological and gene expression alterations in rat penile tissue without impairing erectile function. Journal of Sexual Medicine. 2013;10(12):2952-2966

[87] Kovanecz I, Gelfand R, Masouminia M, Gharib S, Segura D, Vernet D, et al. Oral Bisphenol A (BPA) given to rats at moderate doses is associated with erectile dysfunction, cavernosal lipofibrosis and alterations of global gene transcription. International Journal of Impotence Research. 2014;26(2):67-75

[88] Aversa A, Fittipaldi S, Francomano D, Bimonte VM, Greco EA, Crescioli C, et al. Tadalafil improves lean mass

and endothelial function in nonobese men with mild ED/LUTS: In vivo and in vitro characterization. Endocrine. 2017;**56**(3):639-648

[89] Spitzer M, Bhasin S, Travison TG, Davda MN, Stroh H, Basaria S. Sildenafil increases serum testosterone levels by a direct action on the testes. Andrology. 2013;**1**(6):913-918

[90] Kang S, Park S, Kim MJ, Oh SM, Chung KH, Lee S. A sensitive and selective LC-MS/MS analysis coupled with an online sample enrichment technique for H295R steroidogenesis assay and its application in the investigation of the effect of sildenafil on steroidogenesis. Analytical and Bioanalytical Chemistry. 2013;**405**(29):9489-9496

[91] Andric SA, Janjic MM, Stojkov NJ, Kostic TS. Sildenafil treatment in vivo stimulates Leydig cell steroidogenesis via the cAMP/cGMP signaling pathway. American Journal of Physiology. Endocrinol and Metabolism. 2010;**299**(4):E544-E550

[92] Yigitaslan S, Ozatik O, Ozatik FY, Erol K, Sirmagul B, Baseskioglu AB. Effects of tadalafil on hemorrhagic cystitis and testicular dysfunction induced by cyclophosphamide in rats. Urology International. 2014;**93**(1):55-62

[93] Janjic MM, Stojkov NJ, Bjelic MM, Mihajlovic AI, Andric SA, Kostic TS. Transient rise of serum testosterone level after single sildenafil treatment of adult male rats. Journal of Sexual Medicine. 2012;**9**(10):2534-2543

[94] Mostafa T, Rashed LA, Kotb K. Testosterone and chronic sildenafil/tadalafil anti-apoptotic role in aged diabetic rats. International Journal of Impotence Research. 2010;**22**(4):255-261

[95] Santi D, Granata AR, Guidi A, Pignatti E, Trenti T, Roli L, et al. Six months of daily treatment with vardenafil improves parameters of endothelial inflammation and of hypogonadism in male patients with type 2 diabetes and erectile dysfunction: A randomized, double-blind, prospective trial. European Journal of Endocrinology. 2016;**174**(4):513-522

[96] Jiang T, Zheng L, Su XM, Peng JQ, Sun DC, Li QL, et al. Long-term testosterone supplementation is useful for ED with testosterone deficiency. Asian Journal of Andrology. 2013;**15**(5):699-700

Chapter 4

Non-polymeric Microspheres for the Therapeutic Use of Estrogens: An Innovative Technology

Salvador Espino y Sosa, Myriam Cortés Fuentes,
Jacobo Alejandro Gómez Rico and Manuel Cortés Bonilla

Abstract

Non-polymeric microspheres are stable-shaped particles constituted by crystalline organic compounds. This technology allows controlled release of parental products that has its prime value on estrogen therapy. The structure is a non-polymeric crystalline microsphere that uses a low solubility fatty acid, cholesterol as a carrier. Cholesterol is a waxy lipid, a substance that is insoluble in water and has been recognized as safe as excipient by FDA for the manufacturing of drugs. Cholesterol is a lipid present in the cell membrane and subcellular organelles of tissues and serves as the building block for all steroid hormones including cortisol, aldosterone, estrogen, and testosterone; therefore, this fatty acid provides better biocompatibility than polymers. The use of cholesterol as a low solubility carrier was used to develop a first of its kind, parental HT product for the management of menopausal symptoms carrying estrogen microspheres in an aqueous suspension, which would allow an extended estrogen release maintaining plasmatic therapeutic concentrations. Estradiol doses would be up to 30 times lower than that provided by oral and transdermal routes fulfilling current recommendations regarding the use of a low dose and the nonoral route. Both intramuscular monthly administered formulations of E/P non-polymeric microspheres had favorable pharmacokinetic and safety profiles, suggesting this route as an interesting, novel, and suitable way of treating menopause-related symptoms.

Keywords: hormone therapy, estrogens, technology, non-polymeric microspheres, cholesterol

1. Introduction

1.1 Estradiol pharmacokinetics

In a classic study, the maximum concentration (Cmax) of estradiol at steady state was 161.54 and 98.82 pg/mL and reached at approximately 6 h after a single IM injection of 1.0 and 0.5 mg of estradiol, respectively. Estradiol concentrations decreased through day 4. At day 8, estradiol mean plasma concentration was between 20 and 30 pg/mL and remained stable through day 30. These concentrations are equivalent to those found naturally occurring in early follicular phase of menstrual cycles (31 pg/mL median) in premenopausal women. The estradiol elimination kinetics, based on EC MS, is biphasic, in which the elimination phase (a) presents a mean elimination half-life of 1.34–1.57 days and the second elimination phase (β) a mean elimination half-life of 12.22–16.78 days. Estradiol concentrations remained above 10 pg/mL during the 28 days of interval administration (**Figure 1**) [1].

The safety and effectiveness in menopausal symptoms treatment have been a primary goal in the last decades [2]. Microsphere technology uses of cholesterol as a carrier substance, and the IM administration allows for doses of estradiol up to 30 times lower than those delivered by the leading oral and transdermal alternatives [3].

Due to this delivery system, which allows for an unmatched bioavailability of the active ingredients, non-polymeric microspheres provide comparable or improved efficacy outcomes than seen in the leading high dosage alternatives. At the same time, its low dose formulation results in a superior safety profile compared to other products [4].

Injectable slow release products allow for the formation of crystalline structures in the shape of microspheres, which use cholesterol as a carrier instead of the more commonly used polymers. Cholesterol NF, an inactive ingredient approved by the US Food and Drug Administration (FDA) for use in pharmaceutical specialties—including parenteral products, is generally considered safer than polymers. The highest proportion of cholesterol accepted within a parenteral pharmaceutical product is 5.2% (52 mg/mL); pharmaceutical alternatives that use this technology often contain 0.142% of cholesterol (1.42 mg/mL).

Today, HRT is coming under increasing public scrutiny as hormones in higher dosages are suspected of triggering certain forms of cancer, breast cancer; however, reduced dosages of estradiol are lowering these risks [5].

Millions of women entering menopause suffer from the well-known symptoms but are concerned that the benefits of currently available hormone replacement therapy (HRT) may not justify the suspected risks. Doctors have been looking for alternatives to HRT, such as phytopharmaceuticals, but have found them unsatisfactory in relieving menopausal symptoms [5–8].

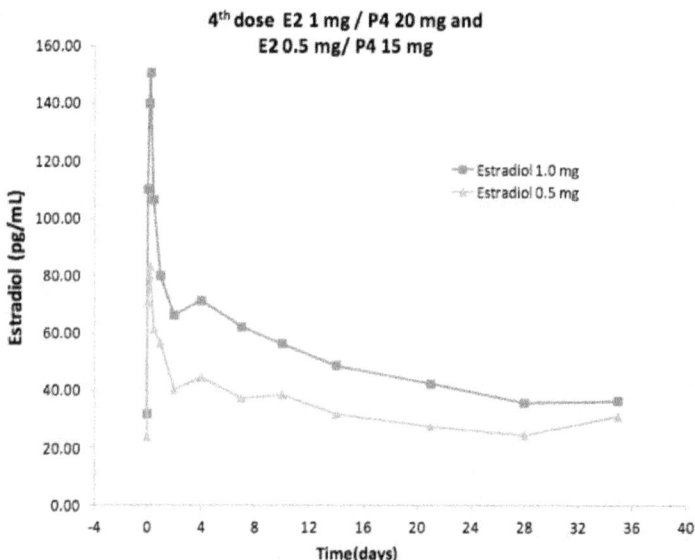

Figure 1.
Estradiol serum profile. Monthly parenteral route of administration.

A safe but effective alternative should be embraced not only by the medical community but also by the millions of women who suffer from menopausal symptoms [3, 9].

The hormonal transition process may last up to 10 years, with 3–4 years being average. Approximately, 50% of women who enter menopause suffer from menopausal symptoms (hot flushes, excessive sweating, sleep disorders, weight increase, nausea, fatigue, irritability, depression). Because these symptoms can so often be debilitating, women are inclined to seek treatment [6].

Treatments can be grouped into three classes:

1. Hormonal treatments, most commonly available as a combination of an estrogen and a progesterone, or estradiol or other estrogens alone (for women who have had a hysterectomy).

2. Nonhormonal treatments:

   a. medicines of natural origin, that is, herbal remedies such as *Cimicifuga racemosa* (leading product: Remifemin), Agnus castus; and soy and red clover isoflavones; and

   b. antidepressants.

3. Traditional remedies: herbal teas, dietary measures, etc.

While the therapeutic efficacy of hormonal therapies has been proven, their use has declined due to perceived and real, safety concerns. It should be a convenient, effective, and low dose product that also addresses the safety concerns relevant to healthy women undergoing menopause [10].

2. Stable-shaped particles of crystalline organic compounds

This technology allows the controlled release of parenteral products and consists of the formation of crystalline arrangement in spherical particles, which use a low solubility excipient as a carrier instead of polymers. Cholesterol is a waxy type of lipid, a substance that is insoluble in water and has been recognized as safe as excipient by FDA for use in the manufacture of drugs and is also a lipid present in the cell membrane and subcellular organelles of tissues and serves as the building blocks for all steroid hormones, and the use of cholesterol gives better biocompatibility than polymers.

The technology used for modification of the release of steroids has been applied in the development of products for the hormonal treatment of the climacteric symptoms (vasomotor symptoms such as night sweats, hot flushes, insomnia, memory loss/forgetfulness, mood swings), providing the clinician with an increased range of options in HRT.

2.1 About the technology

It is well known that many pharmaceutical actives are susceptible to crystallize in different manners, depending on the conditions under which they are crystallized. The polymorphs or pseudopolymorphs are crystalline structures that resulting from crystallization of a substance. When the polymorphs are melted and cooled rapidly below their melting point, that is, melt-congealed, the atoms or molecules forming most substances need some time to arrange themselves in the order most natural for the environment in which they are placed. Therefore, they remain in unstable amorphous or semiamorphous states or organize into metastable polymorphs.

Metastable polymorphs may be enantiotropic, and they can exist in more than one crystalline form. The molecular arrangement can diverge, such that one form is stable above the transition-point temperature and the other is stable below it. As a result, the crystal habit is dynamic and reversible depending on ambient conditions [11].

A natural process that suffers the metastable polymorphs is the "aging," it is a natural crystallization process that occurs over time, transforming the metastable polymorphs into a more stable structure without human interference [12]. In the case of pharmaceutical manufacture, said process is usually costly, lengthy, unpredictable, and dangerous. This is due to the interference of various factors [13].

It is important to consider the time at which the crystallization of metastable particles occurs due to which it can be deformed or destroyed in short time, for example, hours, impacting in the bioactivity and/or bioavailability of crystallized substances. We must be careful with the different dissolution rates of distinct polymorphs of a substance, which can produce loss of uniformity and stability between the batches of the same drug.

When a compound is administered, we often require suspension in an aqueous solution suitable for injection that should not overlook the stable crystallization [14].

When a compound is administered to a patient, said compound is subject to biological fluid that contains water, even before this compound is suspended in an aqueous medium.

In the case of pellets and implants, which are placed in the body at the time of surgical procedures, the previous also applies.

Thereof to achieve full crystallization of substance prior it is administered, it is necessary to assure the physical integrity of the shaped particles and uniformity in the release of the active principle.

With the purpose of improving the stability of therapeutic compounds, some researches have induced the crystallization of them, using a dispersion drying method with temperature being controlled (Matsuda et al. [15]).

Further solubility should consider the shape and size of the therapeutics particles, due to the dissolution of a solid that is also related to the surface erosion [16].

The preservation of the shape and particle size, independently of the form in which a compound is administered either as a solid or as a suspension, is an important factor that assures the control and reproducibility of the bioavailability and biodynamics of the substance. Considering it, Kawashima et al. used two insoluble solvents for spherical crystallization of Tranilast and heat for the conversion of the resulting polymorphs of the process. Some experiments reported that the heat can accelerate the natural process of aging.

In some cases, the integrity or form of the substance could be seen compromised due to the heat requirements. Even though the reproducibility and stability is possible, the size control within the particles of the microspheres can be affected by the use of heat within the experiments.

The heat is also an important factor that can prevent reaching the desired stable polymorph of a specific substance, because in several cases, a hydrate is the most stable polymorphic form and the heat can dehydrate it. In the case of mixtures, the heating for stable crystallization is not recommended. Although the aging process is inferior to the heat method for obtaining stable polymorphs, it is also safer and has fewer limitations.

Among the studies carried out to induce crystallization of polymeric species that use solvent vapors, we highlight the putative crystallization, as well as the change in the mechanical properties of polymeric compounds. To transform a polymer matrix, Pr4VOPc dye (vanadyl phthalocyanine having four propyl substituents), from glassy phase I to crystallized phase II, and organic solvent vapors [17] also have been used.

Tang et al. used organic solvent vapors.

2.2 Characteristics of the technology

The crystalline organic compounds might be formed by homogeneous particles of a single organic compound, or well, they might be formed by mixtures of two or more organic compounds. In aqueous suspension, it is normal that during prolonged storage, the stable particles preserve a constant shape and size. Its features are particularly essential and advantageous in pharmaceutical formulations, due to which stable particles can be fabricated to a uniform size and shape, retaining said characteristics despite of the long-term storage.

The process involves exposure to an atmosphere saturated with solvent vapors, the shaped particles above mentioned, so that one or more organic compounds are in a crystalline, amorphous, or metastable form. Of the liquids used as solvents, at least one or more organic compounds must be soluble.

Among benefits offered by process, it is found that it may be applied to hydrates, which are the most stable polymorphs. Its stability allows the integration of water molecules to crystalline web during formation, since said polymorphs will not drive off water molecules. Due to its susceptibility to high temperatures, the process is also applicable to thermolabile substances. With the exception of the compositions of mixtures-eutectic, a great variety of mixtures involved in the formation of stable structures could not be achieved by means of a process involving heat.

This leads to the utilization of a method that involves crystallization or recrystallizing of an amorphous or metastable crystalline organic compound or mixture. The method consists of the following steps:

1. exposing said compound or mixture to an atmosphere saturated with the vapors of one or more liquids, at least one of which must be a solvent for said compound or mixture, for a time sufficient for transforming the metastable compound or mixture to a stable, crystallized compound, or mixture; and

2. recovering the stable, crystallized compound or mixture for storage or use.

To carry out the process, any container can be used where they can manipulate the different variables, such as volume, pressure, temperature, and atmospheric content. The desired solvent vapors can be contained in a chamber with atmosphere saturated. Once the vapors fill the chamber without causing condensation on the surfaces of the chamber or the particles, the saturation point is reached.

The particles formed preferably acquire shapes of microsphere, pellet, or implant. Although it can be affected by melt-congealing, these are the preferred shaped particles that have uniform and reproducible surface area. The particles formed are usually configured to obtain a uniform particle size or range of sizes. Any process is susceptible to be used as long as it achieves a metastable crystalline conglomeration. The said methods should consider the crystallization of a mixture, and the mixture may be eutectic or noneutectic.

To be exposed to solvent vapors, the particles should be placed in the chamber or some other suitable container; however, said particles should not be immersed or in contact with any other liquid solvents. Once in the chamber, the particles are in a stationary or mobile state.

Depending on the consistency with the established principles, the optimal time necessary to carry out the crystallization will vary, that is, the physicochemical characteristics of the substances, such as size of the particle, the chemical makeup of the particle, the form of the solid state of the particle (i.e., amorphous, metastable crystalline), the type and concentration of solvent used, and the temperature of the treatment. These physicochemical properties will determine if the crystallization process requires seconds or even hours (normally 1–40 h are required, preferably, 1–36 h). A 24-h exposure time seems to be effective. The time ranges do not seem to be modified by the previous partial crystallization of the particles. Other important characteristics that also impact on the optimization of the exposure time of the substance and therefore on the crystallization of it are the solvent system used by the organic compound(s) to be crystallized.

As mentioned above, one of the main advantages of the process is that it can be applied to thermolabile substances, which are susceptible to high temperatures, which exactly what is sought is to avoid them. Thus, particular compound is what will define the applicable temperature range used in the process. To obtain vaporization of the solvent, it is sufficient that the temperature of the vapor in atmosphere is below the melting point of the particles.

The process requires the use of any agent classified as a solvent for the organic compound of interest. Therefore, the latter will determine the selection of the solvent. Among the conventional liquid solvents used in the laboratory are the following examples: water, alkanes, alkenes, alcohols, ketones, aldehydes, ethers, esters, various acids including mineral acids, carboxylic acids and the like, bases, and mixtures thereof. Methanol, ethanol, propanol, acetone, acetic acid, hydrochloric acid, tetrahydrofuran, ether and mixed ethers, pentane, hexane, heptane, octane, toluene, xylene, and benzene are some specific exemplary solvents. Water is an especially useful component of a solvent/liquid mixture, particularly where the most stable polymorph of a substance is a hydrate. Generally, solvents suitable for conventional liquid recrystallization of the compound of interest are suitable as a solvent in the present method.

The compound(s) of the stable particles include any organic compound capable of existing as a crystalline solid at standard temperature and pressure. The stable crystalline solid is formed by particles that are comprised by one or more organic compound(s). The said stable crystalline solid is a lattice of discrete organic molecules, i.e., nonpolymeric.

In the process, those organic compounds having some pharmacological or therapeutic activity are preferred. Even more preferred are the pharmacological compounds susceptible to the formation of polymorphs. These include particles comprised of a steroid or sterol, either, estrogen, androgen and progestogen, such as, 17P-estradiol, testosterone, progesterone, cholesterol, or mixtures thereof. Some nonsteroidal components that can be included in said mixtures are oxatomide/cholesterol, nifedipine/cholesterol, and astemizole/cholesterol.

The particles can be stored in liquid suspensions such as aqueous media, or administered directly to the patient. Due to stabilization of particles of amorphous or metastable crystalline organic compounds, the particles can be stored in liquid suspension, such as aqueous medium, or administered directly to a patient.

2.2.1 Stable-shaped particles of one or more allotropic molecular organic compounds

Allotropic organic compounds can assume two or more distinct physical forms (e.g., different crystalline forms or an amorphous versus a crystalline form). The polymorphs or polymorphic species are allotropic species.

It is important to consider the pharmaceutically acceptable excipients, stabilizers, and buffers, which conform shaped particles and contribute to the stable storage of them.

Among the advantages of stable-shaped particles is the combination of physicochemical properties. First, the particles are configured into desired shapes by means that might not result in the most stable crystalline form of the constituent organic compound. In the solid state crystallization process, the organic compound will assume the most stable crystalline structure, facilitating the retention of the size and shape of the original particle.

A configured particle that comprises of one or more molecular organic compounds, each one which has a uniform crystalline character and possessed of a high degree of storage stability, is the resultant product.

There are several characteristics that lead to the particular predictability and consistent bioavailability and associated biodynamics, such as, the combination of the uniformity of size and shape of the particle and the uniformity and stability of the crystalline structure of the constituent organic compound.

The particle size and the shape of microspheres are prefabricated to desired conditions. Thus, the particles are subject to a solid-state crystallization process that stabilizes the compounds of the particles without loses the size and shape with which they were manufactured.

The resulting particles have greater uniformity of size and shape, more uniform and predictable dissolution profiles, and greater storage stability in various forms, e.g., in liquid suspension such as aqueous media or other storage liquid, as lyophilized solid, or alone as a powder or dry solid. By storage stability, it is meant that the particles have improved shelflife without the loss of their desired uniformity in size and shape, per se. That is, if the desired particle shape is a microsphere, the particles will retain a spherical shape of constant size over periods exceeding several years.

Here, storage stability refers to retention of the original size and shape of the particle, as well as the pharmacological activity of the active agent over a period of at least one .

The technology also involves a method of crystallizing shaped particles of a metastable compound or mixture of compounds without dissolution of the particle and loss of the desired shape.

The crystallization process is affected by exposing said particles to a controlled atmosphere saturated with the vapors of a solvent or solvents. The atmosphere is optionally modified in other respects, for example, pressure, temperature, inert gases, etc. Preferably, the controlled atmosphere is saturated with a solvent vapor but not so much as to effect condensation of said solvent.

More particularly, the method affects crystallization of an amorphous or metastable organic compound in a shaped particle without alteration of the dimensions (e.g., size and shape) of said particle which comprises of: (i) exposing said shaped particle to an atmosphere saturated with the vapor of a liquid, said liquid being a solvent for said organic compound and (ii) recovering said shaped particle wherein the said organic compound is of a uniform crystalline structure.

Alternatively stated, the method involves effecting a solid-state crystallization of a molecular organic compound in a particle of definite size and shape comprising of: (i) exposing said particle to an atmosphere saturated with a solvent for said organic compound; and (ii) recovering said particle, wherein said organic compound in said recovered particle is of a uniform crystalline structure and said recovered particle has retained said size and shape. Retaining the size and shape of the particle is meant to include minor variations in the dimensions of the particle, for example, no more than about 15%, preferably, no more than about 10%.

This technology provides a means for fabricating particles of desired dimension without regard to the resulting allotropic form of the organic compound. After the particle is fabricated into the desired shape and size, the solid state crystallization can be affected to crystallize the organic compound into a storage-stable solid state of uniform crystal structure. Moreover, the solid state crystallization can be affected on particles composed of more than one allotropic organic compound.

Preferably, the shaped particle is a microsphere, and, as a result of the present process, the organic compound(s) of the microsphere are ordered into a single, homogeneous crystalline form without any deterioration in the size or shape of the microsphere.

The term "crystallization" refers to a process by which the most stable polymorph of a particular substance is achieved. Recrystallization refers to a process similar to crystallization except that the organic compound of the particle, rather than being amorphous, was initially only partially crystalline, with a mixed crystalline habit, or crystalline, but of a less stable form. Unless indicated otherwise, the term crystallization includes recrystallization.

The term "solid state crystallization" refers to a crystallization process that is affected without macroscopic dissolution of the compound being crystallized. As used herein, solid state crystallization includes a crystallization process wherein an organic compound within a shaped particle is crystallized or recrystallized by exposure to a solvent vapor without loss or alteration of the shape or size of the particle. It will be appreciated by those skilled in the art that while subtle intermolecular changes will be affected by such crystallization (e.g., creation or rearrangement of crystal lattice structure), the microscopic and/or macroscopic dimensions of the particle will not be appreciably altered. The term "saturated" when used in reference to the atmosphere wherein the crystallization is conducted means that the atmosphere within the chamber or enclosure used to hold the solvent vapors contains the maximum quantity of said solvent in the vapor phase without affecting visible condensation on surfaces within the chamber. Condensation does not include microscopic condensation on the surface of the particles that does not affect their shape.

The term "solvent" refers to a liquid at standard temperature and pressure, and one capable of solubilizing an appreciable amount of a specified solid solute. The solid solute will be a particular organic compound. Solids vary from 0 to 100% in their degree of solubility [18].

A liquid will be a considered a solvent with respect to a particular solid solute provided the solute is at least 10% soluble in said liquid.

The term "particle" refers to a discrete collection of a plurality of molecules of one or more organic compounds. As used herein, a particle may be an ordered collection (e.g., crystalline) or disordered collection (e.g., amorphous) of molecules, or any combination thereof. The term embraces, among other things, microscopic as well as macroscopic particles such as powders, microspheres, pellets, implants, and the like.

Preferably, particles are made of microspheres. The preferred microspheres range in size from 1 micron to 1 mm, more preferably 1 to 500 microns, and most preferably in the range of 1–100 microns, particularly for human use. When the particles are in pellet form, such particles are normally but not necessarily cylindrical with lengths of 1000–5000 microns and diameter of 500–1000 microns. These particles can have important applications for veterinary use and are not injected but deposited under the skin.

The size and shape of the particle will depend on the intended application and the constituent organic compound(s). For example, microsphere size is chosen for practical reasons, that is, a size appropriate for administration using a hypodermic needle or for assuring a desired rate of dissolution.

The term "molecular organic compound" refers to an organic compound existing as stable discrete molecules (i.e., nonpolymeric) and when combined with a plurality of identical molecules, it is capable of assuming one or more ordered crystalline structures. Thus, a molecular organic compound is meant to distinguish from a polymeric species.

The term "metastable" means a pseudoequilibrium state of a solid substance where the content of free energy is higher than that contained in the equilibrium state. A "stable" substance or particle has a crystalline structure whose shape remains unchanged in a standard ambient environment, e.g., in air having varying levels of moisture, for an extended period. However, it should be understood that "stable" does not indicate infinite stability but means sufficiently stable such that the particles remain sufficiently stable for the preservation of their crystalline characteristics during storage and up to their application and use and additionally, after they have been administered to a subject, up to their total dissolution.

The technology also encompasses stable microspheres achieved using the present method. Such microspheres preferably contain a compound having pharmaceutical applications. The microspheres and pellets are useful in human, as well as in animal, therapeutic regimens.

For instance, there is currently a need for compositions that accomplish the sustained release of steroid growth promoters in food animals to promote the growth of such animals. The amount of growth hormone administered to an animal would depend on the particular animal species, hormone, length of treatment, age of animal, and amount of growth promotion desired. The particles can be particularly configured for optimal delivery by injection by varying the particle size.

As discussed above, the microspheres are stable in aqueous fluids and are thus amenable to parenteral injection. Some examples of modes of administration are (IV), intraarterial (IA), intramuscular (IM), intradermal, subcutaneous, intraarticular, cerebrospinal, epidural, intraperitoneal, etc. In addition, the compounds can be administered via an oral route, either as an aqueous suspension or a lyophilized product. Other routes of administration are also acceptable, including topical application, into the eye, or via inhalation in the form of droplets or mist.

The dosage may take the form of a microsphere powder in vials/ampoules, ready to be prepared as suspensions, or take the form of ready-prepared suspensions, packaged into injectable ampoules or directly into syringes, ready to be administered in human or veterinary medicine. The suspension medium may be water, a saline solution, an oil, containing buffers, surfactants, preservatives, commonly used by pharmacotechnicians for preparing injectable substances, or any other substance or combination, which does not threaten the physical and chemical integrity of the substances in suspension and which is suitable for the organism which will receive it. If it is desired to avoid a sudden initial increase in the level of active ingredient in the internal medium of the receiving organism, it will be preferable in the case of ready-for-use suspensions to use liquid vectors in which said active ingredients are practically insoluble. In the case of active substances, partially soluble in the lukewarm liquid vector but insoluble at cold temperature, it is preferable, from the pharmacological point of view, to avoid the formation of precipitates (called "caking effect") by preparing formulations in the form of separate microsphere powder and liquid vector, which will be mixed only at the time of injection.

For most applications in human medicine (duration of action of the active ingredient between a circadian cycle and a menstrual cycle), it is preferable to use microspheres whose diameter is between 5 and 100 microns, depending on the combinations of active substances/carrier substances.

A separation of microspheres according to their diameter may be performed during the manufacturing process using known processes: for example, by cyclonic separators, by sieving using air suction or by sieving in aqueous medium. In practice, it is sufficient if more than 70% of the microspheres have diameters between 70 and 130% of a specified diameter. If necessary, the ideal dissolution curve, determined by the proposed application, may be approached by mixing batches with suitable different diameters. Moreover, particles that do not comply with the specifications may be recycled.

The mechanism by which substances in a solid state crystallize in the presence of vapors containing at least one solvent has not yet been established. The crystallization process may well conform, as regards the effect of the solvents, to the traditional principles that apply in saturated solutions and in molecular mobility.

It is possible that some molecular rotational or transference movement occurs, which seems to depend on the particular type of solvent used and to the temperature of vaporization [19].

.It is clear, however, that the temperatures at which the crystallization is obtained are well below vitreous transition temperatures and are in fact only in accordance with that required for the solvents' vapor pressure. Without wishing to be bound by any theory, we contemplate that the vapor molecules of the solvent or five solvents might form microcondensations and minute accumulations of solvent on the surface of the particles to be crystallized, thus bringing sufficient energy for the surface molecules of the solid particles to form organized structures (e.g., crystalline domains). By the same token, if present in the vapor, water molecules become available for the formation of hydrates, when required for stable polymorphs.

Once the organizational and/or water-absorbing process starts at the surface, it is possible that the crystallization process gradually spreads into the interior of the particle without the need for contact with or dissolution within the solvent. If this is correct, there are two facts, which seem to indicate that these microcondensations or molecular agglomerations, are extremely minute. Firstly, if enough solvent condensation occurred on the surface of the particle, the solvent would at least partially dissolve it and modify its shape. To avoid any partial dissolution, the amounts deposited by the vapor must be extremely minute.

Secondly, during exposure to solvent vapors, the particles, because of their small size and large quantity, inevitably come in contact with one another. If there is any surface dissolution of the particles, as would occur if the substantial quantities of amounts of deposited vapor were not very minute, the particles would tend to stick to each other and form lumps or agglomerates. Under the conditions described herein, this does not occur.

3. Examples

3.1 Example 1: microspheres of 17-beta-estradiol

The spherical 17-beta-estradiol is prepared by spraying at 210°C and solidified at −50°C (spray/congealing method). In this stage, the ME are formed by amorphous solids (**Figure 1**), which when put in contact with water at 40°C, are deformed by the growth of crystals on their surface. In order to obtain the microspheres with the thermodynamically more stable crystalline form, a hemihydrate, the spheres are stored in an atmosphere saturated with vapors of a mixture of ethanol: water (50:50), for 4 h at a temperature of 20 and 25°C. Finally, the microspheres are stored at 40°C to remove the solvent (**Figure 2**). At the end of the process, the spheres are stable, since no change in their morphology is observed after being stored in water at 40°C for more than 9 months.

3.2 Example 2: testosterone microspheres

Two polymorphs and two testosterone hydrates are published in the literature, hydrates being thermodynamically more stable. The preparation of the testosterone microspheres has the same preparation steps that were used for the estradiol microspheres. The stabilization or crystallization was made by storing the microspheres in a saturated atmosphere of vapors of a solution of acetone: water (80:20). The physical stability was evaluated by microscopic observation of storage microspheres in water at 40°C; the freshly prepared testosterone microspheres (uncrystallized) were unstable, while the crystallized microspheres were stable for more than 40 days.

3.3 Example 3: progesterone microspheres

The unstable or metastable spherical solids of progesterone are obtained with the same method (spray/congealing) described in the previous examples. Progesterone has two polymorphic forms, form I have a melting temperature of 131°C and form II with a melting temperature of 123°C, of which form I has a thermodynamically most stable structure.

To obtain the microspheres in the most stable crystalline form, they were stored in an atmosphere saturated with vapors of an ethanol solution: water (50:50) at room temperature for 4 h. The crystallization kinetics of the microspheres was studied by thermal analysis (DSC), where it was observed that polymorph II is the crystalline form that is first formed and later transformed into polymorph I, by the vapors of the solvent mixture.

In the crystallized microspheres, no change in their surface was observed after 6 months of storage in water at 40°C.

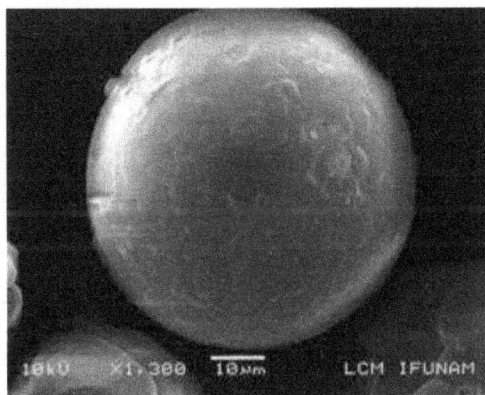

Figure 2.
Estradiol microsphere: estradiol/cholesterol 1:1.

3.4 Example 4: astemizole microspheres

In the same way that the microspheres formed by spheroidal molecules (spray/congealing) are obtained, the microspheres of astemizole are prepared, crystallized with vapors of ethyl acetate or acetone. Its physical stability was confirmed after observing under the microscope spheres stored in water at 40°C for more than 2 months.

3.5 Example 5: astemizole pellets

Pellets obtained in a conventional manner were stabilized with the following crystallization method. When the microspheres were placed in a recipient of approximately 7 L and exposed for 24 h at 20–25°C to the vapors of 2 mL of ethanol kept in a porous cellulose material, the initially amorphous microspheres crystallized completely in the presence of the vapors.

The microspheres were later dried at 60°C in a vacuum for 24 h, and the residual ethanol present in the microspheres was less than 0.01%.

3.6 Example 6: cholesterol microspheres

Cholesterol microspheres were prepared by the spray/congealing method, through microscopic observations of microspheres stored in water, it was concluded that the spheres obtained are formed by amorphous solids.

The crystallization of the spheres is possible by storage in atmospheres of acetic acid at 30°C for 8 h.

3.6.1 Crystallization of substance mixture

The obtaining of spherical particles from mixtures of materials is particularly interesting in the pharmaceutical industry since the end products can have different kinetic (dissolution rates), and chemical (stability) properties to the materials separately. The possibility of stabilizing spheres of material mixtures with this technology greatly increases its application in health areas. To prepare stable spheres formed by mixing of substances, it is important that the materials are thermally stable and chemically compatible.

3.7 Example 7: microspheres of 17-beta-estradiol: cholesterol (40:60)

The microspheres of the mixture were obtained by the spray/congealing method. The stabilization by the crystallization method with solvent atmospheres was possible with the use of 96% by weight ethanol at a temperature of 30°C for 24 h. To remove the solvent, the microspheres were stored in an oven at 60°C. To study the physical stability, the microspheres are stored in water at 40°C and observed under a microscope, after 82 days, the crystallized microspheres retain their spherical shape while those that were not crystallized are deformed by crystals on the surface.

3.7.1 Stability in vivo

In the case of slow release injected or implanted medicinal drugs, the physical integrity of the particles after their administration to the patient is essential to assure the desired rates of delivery and the reproducibility of effect. Thus, the stability in vivo of the microspheres described in the previous example was checked in New Zealand male rabbits.

Microscopy photographs was taken 1, 4, 7 and 14, 10 days after intramuscular injection showed that the microspheres remain whole, until they have finally dissolved. For comparison, microspheres that had not been crystallized were also injected. Their microscopy photographs showed that these microspheres changed into nonspherical shapes.

3.8 Example 8: microspheres of a mixture of 10% 17-beta-estradiol and 90% cholesterol

As for the previous example, the microspheres of this mixture were obtained by melting together the components, sprayed into droplets and congealed into microspheres. Initially, they showed a high amorphous content.

When the microspheres were placed in a recipient of approximately 7.0 L and exposed for 24 h at 0°C, to the vapors of 8 mL of ethanol kept in a porous cellulose material, the initially amorphous microspheres crystallized completely in the presence of the vapors.

The microspheres were later dried at 60°C in a vacuum for 24 h and the residual ethanol present in the microspheres was less than 0.01%.

To evaluate stability of the crystallized microspheres, they were placed in aqueous solution at 40°C and observed by optical microscopy after 141 days.

3.9 Example 9: microspheres of a mixture of 95.2% progesterone and 4.8% 17-beta-estradiol

As for the previous examples, the microspheres of this mixture were obtained by melting together the components, sprayed into droplets, and congealed into microspheres. Initially, they showed a high amorphous content.

When the microspheres were placed in a recipient of approximately 7 L and exposed for 24 h at 20–25°C to the vapors of 2 mL of ethanol kept in a porous cellulose material, the initially amorphous microspheres crystallized completely in the presence of the vapors.

The microspheres were later dried at 60°C in a vacuum for 24 h, and the residual ethanol present in the microspheres was less than 0.01%.

3.10 Example 10: microspheres of a mixture of 60% progesterone and 40% cholesterol

As for the previous examples, the microspheres of this mixture were obtained by melting together the components, sprayed into droplets and congealed into microspheres. They initially showed a high amorphous content.

When the microspheres were placed in a recipient of approximately 7 L and exposed for 24 h at 30°C to the vapors of 2 mL of ethanol kept in a porous cellulose material, the initially amorphous microspheres crystallized completely in the presence of the vapors.

The microspheres were later dried at 60°C in a vacuum for 24 h and the residual ethanol present in the microspheres was less than 0.01%.

4. Conclusion

This technology is widely applicable in forming stable, crystallized particles, microspheres, and pellets of a variety of organic compounds and mixtures that maintain their shape in aqueous solution. Hence, the present method should find significant utility in the manufacture of pharmaceuticals and pharmaceutical compositions, particularly where treatment calls for administration of the pharmaceutical in a slow release formulation. This can be translated into low doses, more secure treatment alternatives, with less frequent side effects, and as an alternative route of administration.

Author details

Salvador Espino y Sosa[1]*, Myriam Cortés Fuentes[2], Jacobo Alejandro Gómez Rico[2] and Manuel Cortés Bonilla[3]

1 Clinical Research Branch, Instituto Nacional de Perinatología, Mexico City, Mexico

2 Centro A.F. de Estudios Tecnológicos (CAFET), Mexico City, Mexico

3 Department of Information Management, Instituto Nacional de Perinatología, Mexico City, Mexico

*Address all correspondence to: manuel.cortes@inper.gob.mx

IntechOpen

References

[1] Newburger J, Goldzieher JW. Pharmacokinetics of ethynyl estradiol: A current view. Contraception. 1985;**32**(1):33-44

[2] New guidelines for the treatment of menopausal symptoms, and the prevention of osteoporosis in women with menopausal symptoms, have been released. Inpharma Weekly. 2004;**1460**:4. https://doi.org/10.2165/00128413-200414600-00006

[3] Stevenson JC. Type and route of estrogen administration. Climacteric. 2009;**12**(sup1):86-90

[4] Cortés-Bonilla M, Bernardo-Escudero R, Alonso-Campero R, Francisco-Doce MT, Hernández-Valencia M, Celis-González C, et al. Treatment of menopausal symptoms with three low-dose continuous sequential 17β-estradiol/progesterone parenteral monthly formulations using novel non-polymeric microsphere technology. Gynecological Endocrinology. 2015;**31**(7):552-559

[5] Li CI, Malone KE, Porter PL, Weiss NS, Tang M-TC, Cushing-Haugen KL, et al. Relationship between long durations and different regimens of hormone therapy and risk of breast cancer. Journal of the American Medical Association. 2003;**289**(24):3254-3263

[6] Nelson HD, Vesco KK, Haney E, Fu R, Nedrow A, Miller J, et al. Nonhormonal therapies for menopausal hot flashes: Systematic review and meta-analysis. Journal of the American Medical Association. 2006;**295**(17):2057-2071

[7] Nahas EAP, Nahas-Neto J, Orsatti FL, Carvalho EP, Oliveira MLCS, Dias R. Efficacy and safety of a soy isoflavone extract in postmenopausal women: A randomized, double-blind, and placebo-controlled study. Maturitas. 2007;**58**(3):249-258

[8] Basaria S, Wisniewski A, Dupree K, Bruno T, Song M-Y, Yao F, et al. Effect of high-dose isoflavones on cognition, quality of life, androgens, and lipoprotein in post-menopausal women. Journal of Endocrinological Investigation. 2009;**32**(2):150-155

[9] The NAMS. 2017 hormone therapy position statement advisory panel. The 2017 hormone therapy position statement of The North American Menopause Society. Menopause. 2017;**24**(7):728-753

[10] Cortés-Bonilla M, Alonso-Campero R, Bernardo-Escudero R, Francisco-Doce MT, Chavarín-González J, Pérez-Cuevas R, et al. Improvement of quality of life and menopausal symptoms in climacteric women treated with low-dose monthly parenteral formulations of non-polymeric microspheres of 17β-estradiol/progesterone. Gynecological Endocrinology. 2016;**32**(10):831-834

[11] Capes JS, Cameron RE. Contact line crystallization to obtain metastable polymorphs. Crystal Growth & Design. 2007;**7**(1):108-112

[12] Yu L. Inferring thermodynamic stability relationship of polymorphs from melting data. Journal of Pharmaceutical Sciences. 1995;**84**(8):966-974

[13] Haleblian JK, Koda RT, Biles JA. Isolation and characterization of some solid phases of fluprednisolone. Journal of Pharmaceutical Sciences. 1971;**60**(10):1485-1488

[14] Kawashima Y, Niwa T, Takeuchi H, Hino T, Itoh Y, Furuyama S. Characterization of polymorphs

of tranilast anhydrate and tranilast monohydrate when crystallized by two solvent change spherical crystallization techniques. Journal of Pharmaceutical Sciences. 1991;**80**(5):472-478

[15] Matsuda Y, Kawaguchi S, Kobayashi H, Nishijo J. Physicochemical characterization of spray-dried phenylbutazone polymorphs. Journal of Pharmaceutical Sciences. 1984;**73**(2):173-179

[16] Carstensen JT. Stability of solids and solid dosage forms. Journal of Pharmaceutical Sciences. 1974;**63**(1):1-14

[17] Tang F, Zhu C, Gan F. Effect of solvent vapor on optical properties of Pr4VOPc in polymethylmethacrylate. Journal of Applied Physics. 1995;**78**(10):5884-5887

[18] Rayne S. Comment on group contribution-based method for determination of solubility parameter of nonelectrolyte organic compounds and solubility parameters of nonelectrolyte organic compounds: Determination using quantitative structure-property relationship strategy. Industrial and Engineering Chemistry Research. 2013;**52**(10):3947-3948

[19] Hancock BC, Zografi G. Characteristics and significance of the amorphous state in pharmaceutical systems. Journal of Pharmaceutical Sciences. 1997;**86**(1):1-12

Bibliographic Review of the Application of Ovulation Synchronization Protocol Based on Gonadotropin-Releasing Hormone (GnRH) and Insulin to Increase the Conception Rate in Crossbred Holstein Cows

Calderón-Luna Joselin and Santos-Calderón Carlos

Abstract

The review work is based on analyzing and recording the effects of the application of ovulation synchronization protocols based on gonadotropin-releasing hormone (GnRH) and insulin for the increase of the pregnancy rate in crossbred Holstein cows in research published between 2013 and 2017. The study was conducted through the integrated search of relevant authors' research using key criteria of both inclusion and exclusion, with results from 244 articles analyzed, where 118 analyzed the interaction of energy balance and ovulation of dairy cows. Fifty-three articles relate the effective ovulation synchronization protocol for the luteal process and 73 articles analyze the effect of insulin in the luteal process; and finally 18 articles are important to address the problem; insulin can be altered as a metabolic hormone by the increase of fat components of the feed ration consumed by cows, thus influencing ovarian function; ovulation synchronization is necessary, which can be based on GnRH and insulin.

Keywords: ovulation, insulin, hormone, GnRH, fertility

1. Introduction

In the present work, the results of the bibliographic study of the published scientific articles are detailed in Journals such as *Boletim Industrial Animal*; *American Dairy Science Association*; *Veterinary (Montevideo)*; *Animal Health Magazine*; *Cuban Journal of Agricultural Science*; *SMVU MAGAZINE*; *Scientific Information System Redalyc*; *Theriogenology*; *Reproduction, Fertility and Development*; *BioMed Research International*; and *Biotechnology Advances* in the last 5 years.

The analysis of the information documents is made based on the references of published works, understanding that they represent the scientific information used in the preparation of various investigations, both to justify and to compare results obtained. The reasons why the authors choose some references and not others are related to several factors. Many of the investigations carried out in the field of the application of the ovulation synchronization protocol, gonadotropin release (GnRH), and insulin use to increase the pregnancy rate of dairy cattle tend to use literature in English in their bibliographical references, with the convinced that this gives more prestige to work. On the other hand, bibliography also selects works published in journals recognized by the main databases, in order to support research that is recognized by the journals that have published them, which obtain, in turn, the databases.

It should be mentioned that follicular growth including the final maturation of the oocyte takes between 8 and 12 weeks in cattle [5]. The metabolites and hormones such as insulin preserves change in concentration in the serum according to the metabolic condition; similarly there is a change following the same pattern in the follicular fluid, although the concentrations may differ [2, 3]. This implies that the oocyte may be exposed to metabolic changes during development and its final maturation.

The majority of high production dairy cows experience a negative energy balance (NEB) in early lactation. The postpartum insemination often occurs around 60 days postpartum so the presumed oocyte for fertilization begins to grow during the dry period before parturition [3, 5].

High and low levels of insulin influence fertility and early embryonic development. The beneficial effects of the different levels of insulin act if the individual is in a state of metabolic homeostasis where the system manages to adapt in response to changes in the energy supply. More studies are needed to get a more complete picture of how insulin concentrations during different reproductive periods correlate with fertility [11].

In addition to increasing the concentration of cholesterol, fat supplementation has increased progesterone plasma concentrations [7, 8, 12, 19, 20]. This has been due to the hypothesis being related to the increase in plasma concentrations of cholesterol, the precursor for steroid synthesis [22].

Intrinsic mechanisms involved are not known in decreased oocyte quality caused by excess energy; some authors have attributed negative excess insulin results because there are changes in the concentrations of other hormones they have studied as IGF-1 and leptin [1]. However, leptin and local growth factors are involved in mechanisms through which diet can affect the quality of oocytes [25]. In addition, adequate concentrations of IGF-I are important for follicular growth and oocyte maturation [10], because excessively bioavailable IGF-I reduces oocyte competition [2].

The objective of this study is to analyze and review the effects of the application of ovulation synchronization protocols based on gonadotropin-releasing hormone (GnRH) and insulin for the increase of the pregnancy rate in crossbred Holstein cows.

2. Materials and methods

The search strategy for the identification of the studies has been divided into three phases:

Phase I. Detailed search in the scientific databases based on the search questions, search strategy, and information sources being the magazines, such as *Boletim de Indústria Animal*; *American Dairy Science Association*; *Veterinary (Montevideo)*; *Animal Health Magazine*; *Cuban Journal of Agricultural Science*; *SMVU MAGAZINE*;

Scientific Information System Redalyc; *Theriogenology*; *Reproduction, Fertility and Development*; *BioMed Research International*; and *Advances in Bioscience and Biotechnology*, to the rest in the search engine, search criteria, and inclusion and exclusion criteria, in the content evaluation criteria (**Table 1**).

Appearance	Explanation
Search questions	• How does the deficiency of luteinizing hormone affect the process of luteolysis?
	• What ovulation synchronization protocol is the most effective for the luteolysis process to be accomplished and to increase the conception rate in crossbred Holstein cows?
	• Is the ovulation synchronization protocol including insulin effective for the luteolysis process to be met and for the conception rate to increase?
Search strategy	• Area: Reproduction of dairy cattle
	• Define the most effective ovulation synchronization protocol including insulin so that the luteolysis process is completed and increases the conception rate
Information sources	• Journals indexed between 2013 and 2017
Search engine	• Google Scholar
Search criteria	• Effect of increase in circulating insulin concentrations
	• Effects of a diet on oocyte
	• Effect of insulin concentrations postpartum period
	• Increase ovulatory response
	• Ovarian response in Holstein cows
	• Energy and its effect on cholesterol
	• Reproductive state of Holstein cattle
	• Formulations of estradiol and progesterone
	• Effect of a single injection of progesterone
Inclusion criteria	• Insulin
	• Effect of preovulatory cholesterol, hormonal profile
	• Deficiency
	• Ovulation
	• Estradiol
	• Progesterone
	• Dairy cows
	• Fertility
Exclusion criteria	• Food, meat, goat, canine, lamb
Criteria evaluation of the contents	• The synchronization of ovulation is an excellent technique to increase reproductive efficiency in crossbred Holstein cows, which favors directly the conception rate, the multiple gonadotropin-releasing hormones shorten the time of the luteal phase in order to increase the fertility of animals, and through insulin induce ovulation, interacting the negative energy balance in this process
Analysis of the information	• Applied method that is more efficient for AI, in Holstein cows
	• Gynecological evaluation periodically to select the best ovulation synchronization protocol and in the same way the most profitable protocol

Table 1.
Search method.

N°	Article name	Authors	Year
1	Effects of supplementation with protected polyunsaturated fatty acids on productive and hormonal parameters of embryo recipient heifers	Juan Camilo Angel Cardona, Harold Ospina Patino, Monica Marcela Ramirez Hernandez, Carolina Heller Pereira*, Kendall Swanson	2016
2	Effects of a high-energy diet on oocyte quality and in vitro embryo production in *Bos indicus* and *Bos taurus* cows	JNS Sales, LT Iguma, RITP Batista, CCR Quintão, MAS Gama, C. Freitas, MM Pereira, LSA Camargo, JHM Viana, JC Souza, PS Baruselli	2015
3	Dry period plane of energy: effects on glucose tolerance in transition dairy cows	S. Mann, FA Leal Yepes, M. Duplessis, JJ Wakshlag, TR Overton BP Cummings, and DV Nydam	2016
4	Manipulation of progesterone to increase ovulatory response	PD Carvalho, MC Wiltbank, PM Fricke	2015
5	Ovarian response and hormone levels in hello cows in different reproductive stages treated with Ovsynch and two progesterone formulations	Cavestany D, Martínez-Barbitta M, Alonzo A, López R, Pilón A, García ME, Segredo A, Sosa N	2016
6	Energy supplementation and its effect on cholesterol levels and preovulatory hormonal profile in cows/energy supplementation and its effect on the level of cholesterol and the preovulatory hormonal profile in cows	Monica Andrea, Moyano Bautista, Carlos Eduardo Rodríguez	2014
7	Metabolic and reproductive state of Holstein cattle in the Carchi region, Ecuador	LR Balarezo, JR García-Díaz, MA Hernández-Barreto, and R. García López	2016
8	Comparison of different estradiol and progesterone formulations	Martínez-Barbitta Ma, González-Guasque Wb, Martínez-Piña Mb, Cavestany Dc	2015
9	Effect of a single injection of progesterone, 5 days	Carlos I. Roque-Velázquez, Hugo H. Montaldo-Valdenegro, Carlos G. Gutiérrez-Aguilar, Joel Hernández-Cerón	2016
10	Relationship between circulating progesterone at timed-AI and fertility in dairy cows	MG Colazo, I. Lopez Helguera, A. Behrouzi, DJ Ambrose, RJ Mapletoft	2017
11	Association between polymorphisms in somatotropic axis genes and fertility of Holstein dairy cows	Lucas Teixeira Hax, Augusto Schneider, Carolina Bespalhok Jacometo, Patrícia M. Attei, Thaís Casarin Da Silva, Géssica Farina, Marcio Nunes Belt	2016
12	Epidemiological evidence for metabolic programming	G. Opsomera B, M. Van Eetveldea, M. Kamala, and A. Van Soom	2017
13	Hypothyroidism reduces the size of ovarian follicles and	J. Rodríguez-Castelán, M. Méndez-Tepepa, Y. Carrillo-Portillo, A. Anaya-Hernández	2017
14	Effects of supplemental dietary energy source	Xueyan Lin, Guimei Liu, Zhengyan Yin, Yun Wang, Qiuling Hou, Kerong Shi, Zhonghua Wang	2017
15	Elevation of blood β-hydroxybutyrate concentration effects	M. Zarrin, L. Grossen-Rösti, RM Bruckmaier, and JJ Gross	2016
16	Single-dose infusion of sodium butyrate, but not lactose, increases plasma β-hydroxybutyrate and insulin in lactating dairy cows	KJ Herrick, AR Hippen	2016
17	The effect of subclinical ketosis on activity at estrus	Andrew J. Rutherford, Georgios Oikonomou and Robert F. Smith	2015
18	Increasing estrus expression in the lactating dairy cow	JA Sauls, BE Voelz, SL Hill, LGD Mendonça, and JS Stevenson	2016

Table 2.
Most important scientific articles.

Phase II. Analysis of the bibliographic citations of the articles selected in the first phase, which are 18 and have been considered of greater importance for the approach of the problem, and are in the range of 5 years for the investigation (2013–2017), same which are reported in **Table 2**.

Phase III. Analysis of the scientific documents published in the journals mentioned in Phase I analyzed their bibliographic citations in phase II.

The search criteria that determine the selection of articles have the words of inclusion and exclusion; similarly, the specific interval of time was selected according to the order of relevance, including patents and citations (**Table 3**).

- Articles on experimental, quasi-experimental studies and studies related to the problem where the effect achieved by applying synchronization protocols based on gonadotropin-releasing hormone (GnRH) and insulin to increase the rate pregnancy in crossbred Holstein cows.

- Studies in which the validity and usefulness of the data are still valid today were analyzed from the 18 scientific articles mentioned in **Table 2**.

Search	Number of results	Specific time interval
Effect of increase in circulating insulin concentrations during the early postpartum period on reproductive function in dairy cow, insulin, reproductive or cattle	24	2015–2017
Effects of a diet on oocyte quality in *Bos indicus* and *Bos taurus* cows, high, or energy "in vitro embryo production"	78	2015–2017
Effect of insulin concentrations postpartum period on reproductive in dairy cow	5	Since 2016
Increase in ovulatory response to the first GnRH treatment manipulation, progesterone, or protocol "first timed artificial insemination," breed	12	Since 2015
Ovarian response in Holstein cows in "different reproductive stages"	4	Since 2015
Energy and its effect on cholesterol level cows supplementation cows energy affect effect preovulatory "hormonal profile "cholesterol-breed	7	Since 2014
Reproductive state of Holstein cattle metabolic energy state deficiency profile, metabolic or profile or bovine indicators, "Holstein cattle," breed	18	Since 2016
Comparison of different formulations of estradiol and progesterone cows or dairy or ovulation or estradiol or progesterone "synchronization of estrus" breed, tropical	3	Since 2015
Effect of a single injection of progesterone on the fertility of dairy cows, insemination fertility, effect on cows, dairy, ovulation, estradiol, progesterone, "after insemination," feed, meat	4	Any moment
Pregnancy rate in Holstein cow pregnancy or rate	11	2017
Treatment of polycystic ovary syndrome with insulin	3	2017
Sources of glucose in ruminants, gluconeogenesis, glucose, lipids, acids	15	2017
Relationship between insulin and present of estrus synchronization artificial protocol or insemination	19	Since 2016
Pregnancy rate percentage in Holstein cows, detection, estrus, insulin, progesterone, estradiol, hormone	41	2017

Table 3.
Search criteria.

3. Results and discussion

Between 2013 and 2017, a total of 597 references were cited in the Bibliography section of the original articles. The distribution by years (**Figure 1**) shows that the highest number of references occurred in 2016 (with 334 references, from 9 articles analyzed) and the lowest figures appear in the years 2013 and 2014 (with 0 and 18 references, from 0 and 1 original work, respectively).

3.1 Language

Eighty-three percent of the references come from documents in English and seventeen percent in Spanish (**Figure 2**). English predominates among the works published in scientific journals mentioned in Phase I.

3.2 Bibliographic analysis of scientific articles

Insulin is a key metabolic hormone that plays a crucial role in the regulation of energy homeostasis in the body [11].

There is a reduction of GHR expression in hepatic tissue in the postpartum dairy cows of high production due to the decrease in blood insulin concentration and negative energy balance (NEB) [20]. Accordingly, the reduction of GH binding in the liver decreases the synthesis of IGF-I. An increase in serum IGF-I is associated with an increase in estradiol production in ovulatory and early postpartum ovulation [4]. Early postpartum ovulation is associated with a shorter birth interval of delivery [21].

It is possible that cows in the semi-extensive system, characterized by lower milk production, are not subjected to a marked NEB. Consequently, these cows are not likely to have a reduction in postpartum GHR liver [20].

The strongly selected for milk yield dairy cows have specific endocrinological characteristics, as low levels of peripheral insulin and low peripheral insulin sensitivity, both contributing to safe guarding glucose milk production. The reverse side of this advanced selection is the high incidence of a wide range of metabolic diseases [15].

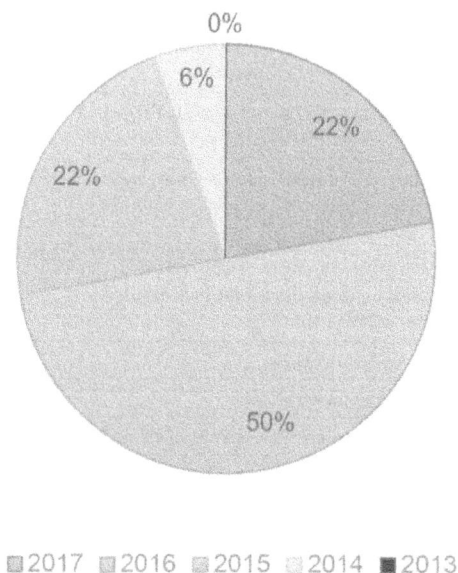

2017 2016 2015 2014 2013

Figure 1.
Distribution of articles by year of publication.

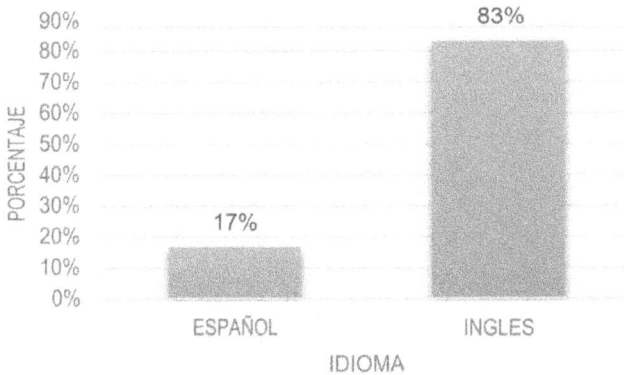

Figure 2.
Language of scientific articles.

Ovarian failure is related with inflammation as well as hypertrophy and visceral adipose tissue dysfunction (VAT). Although hypothyroidism has been associated with obesity, dyslipidemia, and inflammation in humans and animals, its influence on the characteristics of ovarian follicles in adulthood is poorly understood [18].

The source of supplemental dietary energy has variable effects on food intake and lactation performance and intermediary metabolism early lactation in a positive energy balance. The secretion of 5-hydroxytryptamine may be associated with the variable effects of the supplementary dietary energy source.

A higher basal insulin concentration before and after birth. These findings show that the effects of hyperketonemia about plasma glucose concentrations are similar before and after delivery but that endocrine hyperketonemia adaptation differs before and after delivery. B-assume hydroxybutyrate (BHB) is a key metabolic regulator in premature dairy cows and may affect glucose concentration for additional channels as gluconeogenesis and lipolysis altered [26].

Embryo-receiving heifers play an important role in the success or failure of embryo transfer. Some studies have shown positive effects of fatty acids on embryonic development [6, 12, 17, 24] and pregnancy rates [12, 13], which are also positively correlated with higher cholesterol [7, 23] and progesterone [7, 9, 12, 14, 16, 20].

4. Conclusions

The interest awakened from the effect achieved with the application of ovulation synchronization protocols based on the gonadotropin-releasing hormone (GnRH) and insulin to increase the pregnancy rate in crossbred Holstein cows is shown in the increase in publications in the last decade.

The most common strategy to reduce the degree of negative energy balance in early lactation is in reference to the concentration of energy in the diet since it increases the starch or fat components of the ration at the expense of the forage. These strategies alter metabolic hormones, particularly insulin, which can influence ovarian function.

Once the scientific articles have been analyzed applying the relevant methodology, it is concluded that insulin with GnRH may be a protocol that empirically provides benefits, but studies of better methodological quality are still needed to demonstrate the effects attributed to them.

Author details

Calderón-Luna Joselin* and Santos-Calderón Carlos
Higher Polytechnic School of Chimborazo, Ecuador

*Address all correspondence to: natyslu111@gmail.com

IntechOpen

References

[1] Adamiak SJ, Mackie K, Watt RG, Webb R, Sinclair KD. Impact of nutrition on oocyte quality: Cumulative effects of body composition and diet leading to hyperinsulinemia in cattle. Biology of Reproduction. 2005;**73**:918-926

[2] Armstrong DG, Baxter G, Hogg CO, Woad KJ. Insulin-like growth factor (IGF) system in the oocyte and somatic cells of bovine preantral follicles. Reproduction. 2002;**123**:789-797

[3] Britt JH. Impacts of early postpartum metabolism on follicular development and fertility. Bovine Practioners Proceedings. 1992;**24**:39-43

[4] Butler ST, Peltron SH, Butler WR. Insulin increases 17b-estradiol production by the dominant follicle of the first postpartum follicle wave in dairy cows. Reproduction. 2004;**127**:537-545

[5] Butler WR, Beam SW. Energy balance and ovarian follicle development prior to the first ovulation postpartum in dairy cows receiving three levels of dietary fat. Biology of Reproduction. 1997;**56**:133-142

[6] Childs S, Carter F, Lynch CO, Sreenan JM, Lonergan P, Hennessy AA, et al. Embryo yield and quality following dietary supplementation of beef heifers with n-3 polyunsaturated fatty acids. Theriogenology. 2008;**70**:992-1003

[7] Cordeiro MB, Peres MS, Souza JM, Gaspar P, Barbiere F, Sá Filho MF, et al. Supplementation with sunflower seed increases circulating cholesterol concentrations and potentially no on the pregnancy rates in *Bos indicus* beef cattle. Theriogenology. 2015;**83**:1461-1468

[8] Hawkins D, Niswender KD, Oss GM, Moeller CL, Odde KG, Sawyer HR, et al. An increase in serum lipids increases luteal lipid content and alters the misses rate of progesterone in cows. Journal of Animal Science. 1995;**73**:541-545

[9] Hess BW, Moss GE, Rule DC. A decade of developments in the area of fat supplementation research with beef cattle and sheep. Journal of Animal Science. 2008;**86**(Supplement 14):188-204

[10] Landau S, Braw-Tal R, Kaim M, Bor A, Bruckental I. Preovulatory follicular status and diet affect the insulin and glucose content of follicles in high-yielding dairy cows. Animal Reproduction Science. 2000;**64**(3):181-197

[11] Laskowski D, Sjunnesson Y, Humblot P, Andersson G, Gustafsson H, Båge R. The functional role of insulin in fertility and embryonic development—What can we learn from the bovine model ? Theriogenology. 2016;**86**(1):457-464

[12] Lopes C, Scarpa AB, Cappellozza BI, Cooke RF, Vasconcelos JML. Effects of rumen-protected polyunsaturated fatty acid supplementation on reproductive performance of *Bos indicus* beef cows. Journal of Animal Science. 2009;**87**:3935-3943

[13] Lopes CN, Country M, Araújo TP, Oliveira LO, Vasconcelos JL. Efeito mineral suplementação protéica com megalac-e® na taxa of prenhez em primiparous Nelore. Acta Scientiae Veterinariae. 2007;**35**(Supplement 3):970-971

[14] McNeill RE, Diskin MG, Sreenan JM, Morris DG. Associations between milk progesterone concentration on different days and with embryo survival during the early luteal phase in dairy cows. Theriogenology. 2006;**65**:1435-1441

[15] Opsomer G, Van Eetvelde M, Kamal M, Van Soom A. Epidemiological evidence for metabolic programming in dairy cattle. Reproduction, Fertility and Development. 2017;**29**(1):52-57

[16] Peres RFG, Claro Júnior I, Sá Filho OG, Nogueira GP, Vasconcelos JLM. Strategies to improve fertility in *Bos indicus* postpubertal heifers and nonlactating cows submitted to fixed-time artificial insemination. Theriogenology. 2009;**72**:681-689

[17] Petit HV, Cavalieri FB, Santos GTD, Morgan J, Sharpe P. Quality of embryos produced desde dairy cows fed whole flaxseed. Journal of Dairy Science. 2008;**91**:1786-1790

[18] Rodríguez-Castelán J, Méndez-Tepepa M, Carrillo-Portillo Y, Anaya-Hernández A, Rodríguez-Antolín J, Zambrano E, et al. Hypothyroidism reduces the size of ovarian follicles and promotes hypertrophy of periovarian fat with infiltration of macrophages in adult rabbits. BioMed Research International. 2017;**2017**

[19] Ryan DP, Spoon RA, Williams GL. Ovarian follicular characteristics, embryo recovery, and embryo viability in heifers fed high-fat diets and treated with follicle-stimulating hormone. Journal of Animal Science. 1992;**70**:3505-3513

[20] Salas-Razo G, Herrera-Camacho J, Gutiérrez-Vázquez E, Ku-Vera JC, Aké-López JR. Restart postpartum ovarian activity and plasma concentration of lipid and progesterone metabolites in cows supplemented with bypass fat. Tropical and Subtropical Agroecosystems. 2011;**14**:385-392

[21] Spicer LJ, Echternkamp SE. The ovarian insulin and insulin-like growth factor system with an emphasis on domestic animals. Domestic Animal Endocrinology. 1995;**12**:223-245

[22] Staples CR, Burke JM, Thatcher WW. Influence of supplemental fats on reproductive issues and performance of lactating cows. Journal of Dairy Science. 1998;**81**:856-871

[23] Takahashi M, Sawada K, Kawate N, Inaba T, Tamada H. Improvement of superovulatory response and pregnancy rate after transfer of embryos recovered from Japanese black cows fed rumen polyunsaturated bypass fatty acids. The Journal of Veterinary Medical Science. 2013;**75**:1485-1490

[24] Thangavelu G, Colazo GM, Ambrose DJ, Oba M, Okine EK, Dyck MK. Diets enriched in unsaturated fatty acids enhance early embryonic development in lactating Holstein cows. Theriogenology. 2007;**68**:949-957

[25] Webb R, Garnsworthy PC, Gong JG, Armstrong DG. Control of follicular growth: Local interactions and nutritional influences. Journal of Animal Science. 2004;**82**(E. Suppl):E63-E74

[26] Zarrin M, Grossen-Rösti L, Bruckmaier RM, Gross JJ. Elevation of blood β-hydroxybutyrate concentration affects glucose metabolism in dairy cows before and after parturition. Journal of Dairy Science. 2017;**100**(3):2323-2333